RESTORING YOUR CHILD'S MENTAL HEALTH

RESTORING YOUR CHILD'S MENTAL HEALTH

10 INNOVATIVE, DRUG-FREE TREATMENTS

Gracelyn Guyol

Healing Depression & Bipolar Disorder Without Drugs
Who's Crazy Here? Steps to Recovery Without Drugs

Copyright 2018 by Gracelyn Guyol
All rights reserved

ISBN: 0-692-93320-4
ISBN 13: 978-0-692-93320-6

Published in the United States of American by
Ajoite Publishing
4 Exeter Court
Mystic, CT 06355
www.gracelynguyol.com

First U.S. Edition 2018:

Cover design by Heather Rhodes
Studio Petronella

WITH LOVING GRATITUDE

This work is dedicated to my late husband, John T. Guyol. His love and support of 30 years enabled me to find healing and author books to empower others who struggle with mental illness.

CONTENTS

ACKNOWLEDGEMENTS

Heartfelt thanks to the practitioners in this book who provide all-natural treatments that offer realistic hope for recovery from mental disorders. I admire what you do every day and appreciate you taking time to talk with me. Much gratitude goes to Merrin Lazyan for her brilliant editing skills that contributed style and coherence to this effort. I also thank Heather Rhodes for the striking designs and photographs she created at Studio Petronella for this book's cover and my web sites. Working with each of you has been a delightful collaboration.

A Note to Readers

Do not discontinue or reduce your psychiatric medications without the supervision of a holistically-trained medical doctor. Your brain has adjusted to the drugs you are taking, and any change may cause serious reactions and endanger your health.

The recommendations in this book are not intended to replace the services of a mental health professional. Use of this information is the reader's responsibility and it must be utilized in conjunction with medical supervision.

Throughout this text I refer to books, products, web-sites, companies, and practitioners. I do so as a service to readers and do not receive compensation or have financial ties to any of those covered.

Gracelyn Guyol

INTRODUCTION

WHY DRUG-FREE TREATMENTS ARE CRUCIAL

On December 14, 2012, 20-year-old Adam Lanza shot and killed his mother at their Newtown, Connecticut home. He then drove to Sandy Hook Elementary School where he fatally shot 20 children and six adult staff before committing suicide. It was then the deadliest mass shooting at either a high school or grade school, and the third-deadliest mass shooting by a single person in US history. National news coverage focused primarily on gun control. There were proposals for making background-check systems universal, as well as new federal and state gun legislation banning sale and manufacture of certain types of semi-automatic firearms holding more than ten rounds of ammunition.

By January, however, there was still no mention that use of psychiatric drugs had been involved in most major school shootings since 1988. Nor did it mention Adam Lanza was first prescribed Lexapro, a psychotropic drug, and later prescribed Celexa, an antidepressant/anti-anxiety drug, or that he had stopped taking both drugs.

A list of teens committing school violence in the US from 1988-2006 reveals that most shooters were taking psychiatric prescriptions, (primarily antidepressants), according to the Citizen's Commission on Human Rights. Psychiatric antidepressants are well documented as triggering mania, psychosis, hostility, aggression, and suicidal thoughts. Ninety-nine drug regulatory agency warnings have been issued from ten countries and the European Union. Since August 2004, US labels for all antidepressants caution against these and other dangerous side effects. Many experts believe homicidal thoughts should be added to this list of labelled side effects.

David Healy is an internationally respected Professor of Psychiatry at Wales' Cardiff University, researcher, and author of 150-peer-reviewed articles and 20 books. His 2006 study, "Antidepressants and Violence: Problems at the Interface of Medicine and Law," notes the rapid behavioral deterioration triggered by antidepressant use. Using information from pharmacological data and nine criminal trials of violent assaults between 1990 and 2005, his study concludes SSRIs use is directly connected with violence. Healy's book, *Pharmageddon*, is the riveting story of how pharmaceutical companies have hijacked healthcare in America, and how greed has trumped children's safety and long-term health.

In 2011, other researchers revealed additional psychiatric drug concerns. Nancy Andreasen, Editor-in-Chief of the American Journal of Psychiatry from 1993 to 2005, began a long-term study of schizophrenic patients in 1991 that periodically measured brain volumes using magnetic resonance scans. Her results published in 2003 and 2005 noted brain volume reductions but attributed these losses to the disease rather than the treatment. Her 2011 study, published in the February Archives of General Psychiatry, however, drew vastly different conclusions that rocked the mental health community.

Based on MRI scans of 211 schizophrenic patients monitored for 7 to 14 years, she concluded long-term use of antipsychotics and clozapine was definitely associated with brain shrinkage. Brain volume changes were caused by the treatment rather than the disease, said Andreasen, and severity was directly related to dose and length of use.

That same spring, a trio of books from highly credible authors questioned the efficacy of psychiatric drug use. Marcia Angell, MD, former Editor in Chief of the *New England Journal of Medicine,* critiqued all three in the June 2011, *New York Review of Books.*

Psychologist Irving Kirsch's book, *The Emperor's New Drugs,* cites fifteen years of research and meta-analysis of numerous studies, revealing that psychiatric drugs are only slightly more effective than placebos. Psychiatrist Daniel Carlat's *Unhinged, The Trouble with Psychiatry,* unveils the collusion between psychiatrists and pharmaceutical companies, outlining how the profession should be reformed. Award-winning author Robert Whitaker's *Anatomy of an Epidemic* asks why the number of disabled mentally ill in the United States has tripled over the past two decades, despite the touted "improved" treatment of psychiatric medications. He details the harm drugs do, charting how the incidence of mental illness has risen in tandem with their use.

Though they bring different perspectives, all three authors agree on the ineffectiveness and physical damage caused by psychoactive prescriptions. However, none propose what might replace psychiatric drug treatment, which is why this and my two previous books discuss specific, all-natural options that frequently *restore* mental health.

My Healing Education

I became aware of these all-natural treatments during a lengthy personal quest for answers. Diagnosed as Bipolar Type II in 1993, I was prescribed an antidepressant, Wellbutrin, for reducing mood swings. I knew nothing about other options, and my life seemed a little easier, less chaotic.

A year later, my gynecologist discovered I had multiple benign breast cysts and tumors. After surgery to remove all growths, more quickly appeared, which led to a second surgery six months later. Frightened, I consulted a Naturopathic Doctor to help identify the underlying cause of the growths that had appeared so suddenly. She gave me an anti-inflammatory diet (available in Appendix B) and prescribed natural supplements to optimize cellular function. I systematically eliminated all chemical-containing household cleaning, personal care, and lawn care products that might cause cells to mutate. While my energy increased and friends noted my "healthy glow," one new tumor appeared several months later.

Since there had been no cancer in my family and the growths started a year after I began taking Wellbutrin, the drug was finally my prime suspect. I felt it was only a matter of time until a tumor would be malignant. My bipolar symptoms had never been life-threatening, but cancer might be. I tapered off the drug to see what would happen.

Within two months, my new tumor was gone, and all growths stopped. I had eliminated the cause! Yet, I still needed relief for the increasing bipolar symptoms.

Over the next two years, I doggedly pursued drug-free treatments. Finally, a holistic clinic outside of Chicago using an Orthomolecular (meaning "right molecule") medical approach, described in Chapter 10, halted my bipolar manic highs and depressive lows in 2002. Interestingly, the two symptoms had different causes.

The mania was driven by excessively high copper with low zinc and a vitamin B6 deficiency (all due to inherited traits) that ended in just four months of using specific natural supplements. The depression, however, continued for 15 months and was harder to bear without the manic relief.

Clinical trials with bipolar patients, directed by Dr. Andrew Stoll, MD, found therapeutic levels of omega 3 fatty acids in fish oil to be very beneficial. In his book, *The Omega 3 Connection,* Stoll recommended mental patients use 3,000-5,000 mg/day. I was already taking 1,000 mg/day for the anti-inflammatory benefits and had some in the refrigerator. I started taking 1,000 mg with each meal daily. Within 48 hours my deep depression lifted and has not returned.

Tremendously relieved to be free of a horrible, life-impairing illness, I was determined to share what I had learned with others so that they too could experience healing without the use of harmful drugs. (Chapter 1 in my first book has 24 footnoted pages on "Why Drugs Are Not the Best Solution for Mental Disorders.") Patients frequently say, "I hate my meds," and they have many good reasons.

Mild side effects from SSRI antidepressants include dry mouth, drowsiness or insomnia, dizziness, diarrhea or constipation, headache, along with a 30- to 65-pound weight gain. Independent studies find that 54-65% of patients experience sexual dysfunction (manufacturers report only 2-5%). Severe side effects include increased depression and suicidal tendencies, neurologically driven agitation ranging from mild leg tapping to severe panic, tics or muscle spasms, and Parkinsonism. In children, antidepressants also stunt growth, and Prozac and Luvox increase their risk of becoming manic.

It took me three years to write the first book, *Healing Depression & Bipolar Illness Without Drugs* (2006). Lacking any scientific training, I was educating myself at the same time. Each chapter begins with one person's story of halting bipolar disorder or depression, followed by a simplified explanation of the science underlying the treatments that led to recovery. The book brought an invitation to deliver seven-hour, accredited lectures to medical practitioners across the US. I gulped and quickly accepted, spending the next six months preparing. Practitioners were surprised by the science that somehow was missing from conventional medical school training, and they seemed excited to have new, effective treatment options for patients.

After delivering free talks to patients, however, some privately told me they had attention deficit disorder along with the bipolar or depression, making it difficult to read anything lengthy or complex. They asked if I could just tell them what to do to get well, without all the science. My response was a 114-page book covering nine mental disorders: *Who's Crazy Here? Steps to Recovery Without Drugs For ADD/ADHD, Addiction & Eating Disorders, Anxiety & PTSD, Depression, Bipolar Disorder, Schizophrenia, Autism* (2010).

The first half of the book explains the most common *causes* of mental disorders, since there are often several involved. The second half contains individual chapters about each diagnosis listed in the book's title. Diagnosis chapters describe any causes and treatments unique to that ailment. They also contain a bulleted steps-to-recovery list designed for patients to discuss with a medical practitioner trained to use a whole body ("holistic") approach to treatment.

Holistic practitioners make excellent guides because they know that by treating the causes, such as toxic overload, instead of simply medicating each symptom, you can help restore the body's built-in ability to heal. Students entering medical school may choose from one of seven accredited naturopathic universities in the US to become Naturopathic Doctors (ND), who are specifically trained to use only drug-free treatments. Many Medical Doctors (MD) with established practices attend conferences or take classes to add holistic methods (Orthomolecular, Alternative, Integrative, or Functional) into their skill set.

Raising awareness of recovery as a realistic goal when using drug-free treatment options became my life's purpose. Empowering others who suffer from mental illnesses was (and still is) the most emotionally satisfying work I have ever done, which is why I felt compelled to take action following the Newtown shootings.

Connecticut Children's Mental Health Task Force

Upset by the news media's focus on guns, it finally hit me that most journalists do not have the training required to suspect that psychiatric drug use might have led to these shootings. I sent a press release to over 900 health media outlets across the US, titled "Crucial Newtown Shooting Questions Not Yet Asked. What Do School Shooters Have in Common?" I also wrote an article listing the teens who committed school violence from 1988-2006, offering it free to the press. It included the year, name and age of the shooter, which psychiatric drug they had been taking (primarily antidepressants), how many people they had killed, in what state the shooting occurred, and my source.

What did the assailants have in common? Many had begun taking or had abruptly stopped taking psychiatric drugs prior to the attacks; all except one were boys; and all used firearms except one, whose weapon was a knife. The press release also included the "well accepted knowledge" (cited earlier here) stating how psychiatric drugs often cause mania, psychosis, hostility, aggression, and suicidal thoughts, with drug regulatory agency warnings.

No one requested the article. Yet by the following week, many US television news outlets opened their shows by calling for better treatment of psychiatric problems in children.

Encouraged, I sent a letter to the governor offering my knowledge of alternative, drug-free treatments. Within a month I was invited to serve on a new Connecticut Children's Mental Health Task Force, formed to recommend changes to legislators. Each Task Force member served for one year. I was the only one with broad knowledge of "alternative" medicine. For six months I researched drug-free treatments that were scientifically shown to be effective, affordable, and easy for patients to use. In July 2014, I submitted a 30-page executive summary of ten options for Task Force recommendation to the legislature and potential consideration by the four Connecticut agencies serving children who have mental problems.

No changes resulted from my efforts. This was not a big surprise to me. Having worked in major corporations, I knew large, bureaucratic organizations were seldom innovative and often resist change. Still, I was happy knowing I had much of the research completed for my next book—the one you are holding—and that many parents of children in need of treatment would most likely be interested.

Plans for the Future

Early this year I received final approval of my application to start a 501(C)(3) holistic mental health advocacy and educational non-profit: **Mind Energy Innovations, Inc., (MEI).** If after reading my books you want to support raising consumer awareness and expanding use of this approach to treating mental illnesses, please go to https://www.mindenergyinnovations.org and make a tax-deductible donation.

To stay informed about MEI's progress and activities, become a Friend on my Facebook page, "Holistic Healing with Gracelyn." https://www.facebook.com/Holistic-Healing-with-Gracelyn-430514663769926.

May this book provide hope for a brighter future and lead to the ***restoration of mental health*** for your children, friends, and family.

With love and compassion,
Gracelyn Guyol, February 1, 2018

PART I

QUANTUM HEALING

CHAPTER 1

HOMEOPATHY'S "NEW" NANOPARTICLES
FOR ALL MENTAL DIAGNOSES

Homeopathy, a medical treatment created more than 200 years ago, is now used by over 500 million people on a regular basis. According to the World Health Organization, it is the largest complementary and alternative medicine utilized globally, no doubt due to its low cost, safety, and effectiveness. Consistent improvements to medical problems treated with homeopathic remedies have resulted in them being covered by national health systems in 42 countries. Yet among the 324 million residents of the United States, many of whom struggle to pay for medical insurance and prescriptions, only six million people use homeopathy, and those who do *must pay for it out-of-pocket.*

The story behind this is interesting, with the beginning told best in a remarkable and delightful book, *Impossible Cure, The Promise of Homeopathy*, by Amy Lansky, PhD. In it, Lansky interweaves details of how homeopathy cured her son's Autism with the history of Christian Frederich Samuel Hahnemann's creation of a new medical system during the 1790s.

Christian Frederich Samuel Hahnemann

Fluent in nine languages, Hahnemann began studying medicine at age 20 in Germany and translated scientific texts for income. Nine years later he abandoned the medical practices of his time—induced vomiting, diarrhea, bleeding, and using opiates or toxic doses of mercury—and adopted the teachings of Hippocrates, a Greek physician born in 460 BC. Considered the father of

3

modern medicine, the Hippocratic oath, "First do no harm," is still taken by many graduating doctors.

Hippocrates maintained healing could be achieved in one of two ways: through the action of "opposites" (using a medicine that creates the opposite effect of the patient's symptoms) or through the action of "similars" (using a medicine that creates in a healthy person the same symptoms experienced by the patient). Hahnemann had studied Hippocrates writings, as well as that of Paracelsus and other medieval alchemists, and knew they had achieved cures using the latter approach.

Hahnemann became well-known and sought after for his translations of important medical texts. Yet he continued searching for a better method of healing that made sense scientifically and consistently worked. William Cullen, professor of medicine at the University of Edinburgh and author of *Treatise on Materia Medica*, hired Hahnemann to translate his book. In it Cullen described using a Peruvian bark called *cinchona* or *china*. The source of quinine, it is still the primary treatment for malaria. However, Cullen's explanation of how *cinchona* facilitated healing—that it had a tonic effect on the stomach—did not make sense to Hahnemann.

He decided to test *cinchona*, and systematically took overdoses of the bark for several days, recording his reactions. His notes summarize symptoms that are typical of an intermittent fever that lasted three hours every time he repeated the dose. Yet when he stopped taking the medicine, he returned to good health. This experience convinced Hahnemann that the "similars" principle could become the foundation of a new medical system.

Hahnemann's "Law of Similars" states that a substance which causes symptoms similar to those of a disease state can cure a sick person of that disease. Unlike others who utilized the principle occasionally, he decided to explore it to the limits. He tested hundreds of substances for responses, calling them "provings." It became his life's work and the basis of homeopathy.

Homeopathic Remedies

Homeopathy grew rapidly for the simple reason it was more successful than most 19th century medicines. The American Institute of Homeopathy, founded in 1844, was the first medical association of any kind in the United States.

By the turn of the century, there were 20 homeopathic medical schools in this country.

The pace of medical discoveries was rapid in the early 20th Century. Several new vaccines were created; the blood typing system was developed; the existence of vitamins and their importance to health were documented; and use of insulin for diabetes began. Yet infected wounds and the tuberculosis and pneumonia bacteria were still notorious killers.

In 1928, Alexander Fleming's accidental discovery that mold on a discarded culture plate at London's St. Mary's Hospital had antibacterial action spurred tremendous excitement for "modern medicine" and launched the use of penicillin.

Gradually, homeopathy use declined in the United States (although not in other countries). The downward spiral was fed by decades of scientific controversy over the high dilution of homeopathic remedies. Utilizing the best biochemical assays of that era, not one molecule of the original bulk substance could be found in the remedies. Thus, many doctors maintained that health improvements must result from a patient's belief in the remedy, known as the "placebo response," not from the substance itself.

Undiluted remedies could bring about a cure, but they could also cause side effects. Hahnemann's ideal form of cure was rapid, gentle, permanent, and reliable. Convinced by the reliability of the Law of Similars, Hahnemann worked to make remedies gentle, easier for patients. He increased the dilution ratio of an active ingredient with water and alcohol, but when too diluted, found there was no effect. He tried to ensure remedies were well-mixed by succussing (vigorously shaking them). Those made by dilution and succussion seemed to have greater curative power. He called the process "potentization" to indicate these enhanced benefits. Even nonmedicinal substances—such as onion, garlic, salt, cinnamon, asparagus, potato, and milk—became powerful remedies following potentization.

Hahnemann experimented with higher potencies as well. He suspected the effects of potentized remedies were unlikely to be biochemical at all but that they acted on a more "energetic" or insubstantial plane – what he called the "life principle" or vital force, what Greeks called *dynamis*, an inherent power.

Thus, Hahnemann spent 40 years refining and improving the remedies, testing new dilutions, methods and repetitions for dosing, along with various avenues of administration. At the same time, he developed additional remedies to expand treatment options. Today there are an estimated 3,500 homeopathic remedies in use.

Enlightening 2009 Discovery

Two centuries after Hahnemann did his important work, Dr. Jayesh Bellare, "Institute Chair Professor" of Chemical Engineering at the Indian Institute of Technology, who also had 20 years of worldwide experience in nanotechnology, proved Hahnemann right.

The argument that homeopathic remedies were merely eliciting a placebo response was still used to disparage these inexpensive treatments. However, the claim had lost credibility because it was widely observed that the remedies worked. This was especially true in India, where 100 million people now depend solely on homeopathy for medical care; thanks to an entire system of homeopathic medical schools and licensed practitioners able to treat in hospital settings.

In 2009, Dr. Bellare observed that homeopathic remedies were manufactured in a process similar to modern techniques for producing nanoparticles. He and colleagues investigated six different commercially made homeopathic remedies using sophisticated electron microscopes and lab tests. Results revealed original source material was present in the remedies in nanoparticle forms at 6C, 30C, and 200C dilutions. Above 12C, no source material should have been present, yet it was—a stunning revelation that quickly broadened scientific interest in homeopathy.

The science of quantum physics explains how nanoparticles work, if you speak that language. I am not fluent, so allow me to share the concise explanation of two experts, for readers who are scientifically curious.

Iris Bell, MD, PhD, is a Board-Certified Psychiatrist who has served on the faculties of Harvard Medical School, University of California San Francisco, and University of Arizona. She is also a researcher in Complementary and Alternative medical areas for 30 years. Bell speaks fluidly about homeopathy on YouTube videos, discussing extremely complex, biological functions in a concise manner. In her 2012 study, "A Model for Homeopathic Remedy Effects," she says:

> "Nanoparticles stimulate hormesis, a beneficial low-dose adaptive stress response. Homeopathic remedies prescribed in low doses

spaced intermittently over time act as biological signals that stimulate the organism's allostatic biological stress response network, evoking nonlinear modulatory, self-organizing change.... Properly-timed remedy dosing elicits disease-primed compensatory reversal in direction of maladaptive dynamics of the allostatic network, thus promoting resilience and recovery from disease."

Professor Marcin Molski, HAB, PhD, MSc, at Adam Mickiewicz University in Poland, has received awards from the Polish Chemical Society in 1992 and 1998, and is Vice-Head of the scientific committee of the Bioelectronics Foundation. Two of his fields of research are theoretical investigation of biological, physical, and chemical properties of substances used in cosmetics and medicine, and non-linear, non-local, coherent and quasi-quantum phenomena in biological systems.

The April 2010 article in *Homeopathy Journal* by Dr. Molski, "Quasi-quantum Phenomena: The Key to Understanding Homeopathy," summarizes the action. Based on first- and second-order Gomperzian kinetics, it has been proved that the crystallization and its reciprocal process of dissolution are classified as quasi-quantum non-local coherent phenomena. This results in formulated ad hoc macroscopic versions of quantum non-locality, entanglement and coherence utilized in interpretation of the homeopathic remedies activity and effectiveness.

Treatment Today

Despite the complicated nanoparticle science, homeopathy remains very simple to use. Treatment begins with the practitioner obtaining a detailed medical history and observing your unique personality, likes and dislikes. Such details enable selection of the specific homeopathic remedy that will best resolve physical and behavioral problems. Classical homeopathy uses only one remedy at a time. Doses can be raised or lowered, or totally new remedies tried, until a positive response is evident. Improvements may occur immediately or take several months or more to achieve maximum benefits, depending on how complex the medical challenge.

What makes homeopathy most appealing to busy patients is that all they need do is take the remedy as directed once a day. Dietary and lifestyle changes are often recommended, but they are not required. If psychiatric medications are currently being taken by a patient, they are continued with the homeopathic remedy until medications are no longer needed.

In the United States, homeopathy cost and availability depend on where you are treated, with higher rates in major cities. For an initial 60- to 90-minute visit with an MD or ND homeopath, $100-300; other homeopaths will charge $50-250 for an initial session; 15- to 45-minute follow-up visits with MD/ND, $50-100; other homeopaths will charge $30-80. Homeopathic remedy costs range $7-25 per bottle or less in kits.

Clinical Trials

Homeopathic remedies are regulated as drugs under the Federal Food, Drug, and Cosmetic Act. They are not currently evaluated for safety or effectiveness, given their 200-years of use around the globe without serious side effects. Hundreds of clinical trials, systematic reviews, and meta-analyses of homeopathic remedies have been conducted over several decades. But until the discovery of nanoparticles in homeopathic remedies in 2009, there was obvious bias against homeopathy in much of the prior research.

A classic example of this bias is the first comprehensive review of homeopathy research, published in the *British Medical Journal* in 1991, that reviewed 105 clinical trials. The authors, three orthodox epidemiologists, came to this conclusion: "The amount of positive evidence even among the best studies came as a surprise to us. Based on this evidence we would readily accept that homeopathy can be efficacious, if only the mechanism of action were more plausible." Fortunately, this argument is now history. Here are conclusions from selected studies, published between 1999 and 2011.

A randomized, double-blind, placebo-controlled trial of 60 mild traumatic brain injury (MTBI) patients was conducted at Spaulding Rehabilitation Hospital. Homeopathic treatment was "the only significant or near-significant predictor of improvement" on the Difficulty with Situations Scale, the Symptom Rating Scale, and Ten Most Common Symptoms of MTBI tests, indicating "clinically significant outcomes" from homeopathic treatments versus controls (Chapman EH, et al, 1999).

The purpose of a prospective trial was to assess homeopathy's effectiveness in hyperactive patients compared to methylphenidate (MPD), a prescription drug given to children with ADHD. One hundred and fifteen kids (92 boys and 23 girls), were included, with an average age of 8.3 years. After treatment for 3.5 months, 75% of children had responded to homeopathy with a clinical improvement rating of 73%. Twenty-two percent of children needed MPD. Researchers concluded, "Where treatment of a hyperactive child is not urgent, homeopathy is a valuable alternative to MPD.... In preschoolers, homeopathy appears a particularly useful treatment for ADHD" (Frei H, Thurneysen A, 2001).

The long-term outcome from homeopathic treatment was studied in 3,981 patients (2851 adults and 1130 children) who were referred by 103 primary care practices having additional specialization in homeopathy in Germany and Switzerland. Ninety-seven percent of all diagnoses were chronic, with an average duration of eight years. For adults and young children, "major" quality of life improvements were observed after 3, 12, and 24 months, but no changes were seen in adolescents (Witt CM, et al, 2005).

Chronic primary insomnia is defined as difficulty initiating or maintaining nightly sleep for a period of at least one month. Thirty participants were selected and divided between homeopathic simillimum treatment and placebo groups, with results measured by their Sleep Diary and Sleep Impairment Index. The Sleep Diary data revealed simillimum treatment resulted in significant increase in duration of sleep, a significant improvement in Sleep Impairment Index scores, and improved responses to all questions, revealing a statistically significant difference between the groups (Naude DF, 2010).

Young adults of both sexes—with above average scores for either cynical hostility or anxiety sensitivity and a history of coffee-induced insomnia—participated in a month-long study. Fifty-four received placebo pellets on night eight and homeopathic verum pellets on night 22, in 30C doses of one of two homeopathic remedies: Nux Vomica or Coffea Cruda. The vernum remedies significantly increased total sleep time and non-REM sleep (Bell IR, 2011).

Ninety-one outpatients having moderate to severe depression participated in an eight-week, double-blind trial that tested the "non-inferiority and tolerability" of individualized homeopathic medicines (Quinquagintamillesmial, also called Q-potencies). Fluoxetine was used as an active control. The primary measure of effectiveness was the mean change in Montgomery & Asberg Depression Rating Scale scores. There were no significant differences between the groups in percentages of response rates, remission rates, or tolerability, although a higher percentage of patients treated with fluoxetine reported adverse side effects. Results indicated the non-inferiority of individualized homeopathic Q-potencies. (Adler UC, et al, 2011)

Because Homeopathy is so safe, inexpensive, easy to use, and effective for 70-80% of patients, it is the first mental health treatment I suggest for children.

Resources:

Amy L. Lansky, PhD, author, *Impossible Cure, The Promise of Homeopathy*, R. L. Ranch Press (2003), www.impossiblecure.com.

Homeopathy and Mental Health Care, Integrative Practice, Principles and Research (Homeolinks Pub., 2010); all chapters are authored by leading homeopathic practitioners around the world, edited by Christopher K. Johannes, PhD, and Harry van der Zee, MD.

Judyth Reichenberg-Ullman, ND, and Robert Ullman, ND, two books: ***Ritalin Free Kids (2013),*** and ***Rage Free Kids*** (2005), which discuss the leading homeopathic remedies for hyperactivity and its various syndromes.

Dana Ullman, MPH, CCH, is certified in classical homeopathy and one of its leading advocates. The author of 10 books, Ullman is founder of Homeopathic Educational Services, a resource center for homeopathic information and correspondence courses, which has co-published over 35 books on homeopathy with North Atlantic Books. For an informative interview of Dana Ullman about using Homeopathy for children, go to https://www.homeopathic.com/Articles/Introduction_to_Homeopathy/Homeopathy_and_Childrens_Health_An_Interview.html

CHAPTER 2

BioEnergetic Assessment and Homotoxicology For All Mental Diagnoses

When I learned that Sheila Reed found healing for her son's Autism through bioenergetic assessment and homotoxicology remedies, I immediately telephoned for an interview. Although I have used homeopathic remedies for minor ailments like poison ivy outbreaks and leg cramps, I wanted to learn more about what sounded like a simple, yet updated method of treatment that could benefit so many children.

A Licensed Clinical Social Worker, Board Certified Holistic Healthcare Practitioner, with a BA in Sociology/Applied Social Relations, Reed also has a BA in Psychology and Masters in Social Work. She now specializes as a bioenergetic and homotoxicology practitioner, treating children and adults from her office in Old Saybrook, CT.

BioEnergetic Assessment

Bioenergetic assessment measures the energetic patterns of each organ and body system using acupuncture points on the hands or feet. The degree of inflammation, degeneration, or level of stress present can be determined and immediately used by the practitioner to create a treatment plan for each individual that helps restore the body's internal equilibrium and innate healing ability.

This bioenergetic approach is based on extensive research conducted in the 1940s by Reinhard Voll, MD, a German medical doctor, engineer, and acupuncturist. Voll was fascinated by the 3,000-year-old Chinese practice of treating patients' ailments by correcting and maintaining proper energy flow, called Qi' (pronounced chee), throughout their body. The practice is now the art and science known as Acupuncture.

Meridians are a network of energy channels that move Qi' throughout the body. While Chinese doctors typically use 12 meridians for healing, there are 21 basic meridians, all having numerous acupuncture "points." Each point is related to a specific gland or functional region found within an organ. This energy system is identical in every man and woman; we all have the same meridians and acupuncture points.

Dr. Voll located and mapped an additional 800 acupuncture points in the human body during his 40 years of research. He also developed a method for testing energy flow, now called Electro-Acupuncture according to Dr. Voll (EAV), or Electro-Dermal Screening, or Meridian Stress Assessment. Documented and proven in over a decade of hospital studies in Germany, the system is used in Europe by over 25,000 medical practitioners. In the US, however, it is primarily used by complementary and alternative medical practitioners.

The EAV system assesses health by measuring energy flow along acupuncture meridians to organs, glands, and the nervous, circulatory, and other body systems. While the systems are physical and chemical in nature, there is also an unseen energetic component in the body's electrical pathways that acupuncturists have utilized for centuries to restore health.

During the 1950s, other investigators found that certain points on the skin consistently had much higher electrical conductance. Normally, skin has resistance of 2-4 Ohms, but at specific classical acupuncture points, a resistance of 100,000 Ohms was consistently found. These came to be known as "information access windows" that reveal the health status of an organ connected to that point.

Computers with specialized software can now measure skin resistance from acupoints in the fascia underneath the skin. To do so, the body becomes part of a "closed circuit," using conductance from two areas. The first point of contact is a ground (negative) electrode the practitioner places in the palm of a patient's hand. At a second point on the opposite hand, a test probe (positive electrode) is placed on the skin over a specific acupuncture point, closing the circuit.

A pre-set amount of electric current flows from the device through the probe. Conductance is measured through the acupuncture point being tested, delivering a value that is an indirect measurement of the "energetic system."

This is not a standard lab test. When the bioenergetic assessment system tests the liver meridian, it is not testing the actual liver but the electrical vibration (also called resonance) of the liver, providing a measurement of its weakness or health.

When Sheila Reed performed a bioenergetic assessment of me, using an Avatar brand computerized system, my resonance showed extremely high levels of lead, along with low levels of mercury and nickel (confirming a "challenge" lab test for metals I had done the previous year). Assessment of other systems confirmed the presence of Candida yeast species; Fluke parasitic flatworms; Epstein Barr and Herpes Simplex virus; Spirochetes and Borrelia Miyamotoi that cause Lyme Disease; the fungus Trichophyton Equinum; a fever-causing bacteria Ehrlichia Sennetsu; and diarrhea-causing protozoan Giardia lamblia. While some of my invaders had been diagnosed and treated in the past, my immune system appeared to be holding everything in check since I had no active symptoms.

After six months of simply placing drops of specific homotoxicology remedies under my tongue every morning and taking two other natural supplements to aid detoxification, reassessment showed the metals and pathogens were gone—even those related to Lyme disease!

BioEnergetic Assessment of Lyme Disease

The treatment of Lyme disease is a powerful example of the benefits of having a bioenergetic assessment and taking homotoxicology remedies. Lyme is an active bacterial infection from the bite of deer ticks (found on every continent except Antarctica), and one strongly linked to psychiatric disorders in adults and children.

Mental and Emotional Symptoms
Connected to Lyme Disease:

Attention Deficit Hyperactive Disorder
Anxiety
Brain fog
Bipolar Disorder

Crying
Decline in reasoning
Depression
Learning disabilities
Memory loss
Obsessive Compulsive Disorder
Rage/violence

A debilitating and sometimes chronic illness, Lyme disease has baffled doctors for decades because it is difficult to diagnose. Blood tests sent to three top medical labs in the US failed to detect 35 percent of Lyme antibodies. Plus, Lyme bacteria can morph into three forms, only two of which are active and symptom-producing. The two active forms release fat-soluble toxins—stored in body fat and fatty brain tissue—that overwhelm and lower immune function, aiding its survival.

The active spirochete form of Lyme bacteria is spiral shaped (enabling it to drill into tissue, organs, bone) with an outer cell wall that is responsible for the initial, rapidly spreading infection. The second active form, a cell-wall-deficient variant having no cell walls of its own, can hide inside body cells, even immune system cells, to avoid detection. A third form is the ultimate stealth device: a dormant ball-shaped cyst that produces no symptoms and is surrounded by an almost impenetrable outer shell that cloaks it. Each of these three forms can convert into one of the other forms to increase the odds of continued existence and the opportunity to replicate.

Soon after a Lyme tick bite is felt or visible, taking a course of antibiotics (with probiotics between doses to maintain beneficial gut bacteria) helps some people halt its development. However, not everyone discovers the Lyme tick or its bulls-eye ring on their skin quickly enough. Doses of antibiotics given too long after infection may simply cause the bacteria to take cyst form until the antibiotics have lost effectiveness, allowing even more aggressive symptoms to unexpectedly return later.

A bioenergetic assessment rapidly identifies a wide variety of toxins and invaders that sap the body's healthy vibrations, as well as those directly causing disease. Homotoxicology remedies are the all-natural medicines used to eradicate these causes. They are based on and made according to the same principles as homeopathy, but with one difference.

Homeopathic remedies utilize only one "active" ingredient in each remedy. Homotoxicology remedies contain multiple active ingredients that can simultaneously address numerous pathogens, toxins, and other Twentieth Century challenges.

Homotoxicology

Homotoxicology remedies link classical homeopathy with biomedicine. They were developed in Germany during the 1930s-40s by Dr. Hans Heinrich Reckeweg, a clinical expert and passionate homeopath. A translation of the 2015 European Partnership for Action Against Cancer report describes his pivotal role in introducing new, pharmacological principles and using several homotoxicology remedies in combination to halt serious, chronic illnesses:

"Today, it is clear the great contribution made by Reckeweg towards medical science: he was able to integrate, in a single vision, the principles of Hahnemann and the new trends of modern medicine. Some modern researchers have defined homotoxicology as "homeopathy of the year 2000," others viewed it as a meeting point between the genius of Hahnemann empiricism, the charming Eastern medical philosophy, and Western science focused on experimentation.

"Homotoxicology has its roots in classical homeopathy but it is linked to pathophysiology and it is used during the diagnosis, while the substances used as therapy are prepared according to the standards of the Homeopathic Pharmacopoeia.

"Inside the pharmacology there is one of the most brilliant aspects of Reckeweg: in addition to classical homeopathic remedies, he introduces a series of "new," pharmacological principles as a result of the interpretation of biochemical and immunological aspects of the diseases; new nosodes appear ranging beyond the diatesis nosodes introduced by Hahnemann, there are the intermediates catlysts of Krebs cycle, the organotherapici suis and the class of compounds prepared. The compounds are an association of remedies whose principle can be summed up in three words: synergy, complementarity, completeness in accordance with the Burgi principle."

The purpose of homotoxicology treatment is not to suppress symptoms but to detoxify the body and repair damage caused by *toxins*. Its use of several remedies to address serious chronic illnesses triggers an effect that activates the body's "reserve defense systems."

From an immune system standpoint, homotoxicology remedies increase a cell-mediated response that does not involve antibodies. But this is not the only reaction. The body's powerful reserve defense response zeroes in on a specific toxin, bacteria, or other pathogen that has been the triggering cause. It can also target anything containing something similar to the cause, even if it is only part of the molecule. Neutralizing targets that merely resemble the original target is crucial, since many pathogens, such as viruses, frequently mutate and change.

Dr. Reckeweg believed diseases are the expression of the body's fight against toxins in order to neutralize and expel them or are an expression of the struggle a body makes to compensate for damage caused by irreversible toxins.

Humans normally excrete toxins through feces, urine, and sweat, provided these systems are not blocked. When the ability to eliminate toxins is compromised, however, the body experiences progressive stages of illness that correspond to the buildup of toxins. The *symptoms of illness* result from the body's resistance to toxins. If symptoms are suppressed with steroids, antibiotics or other prescription drugs, toxins are driven deeper into cells, making a condition more intractable.

For instance, millions of patients are encouraged to take anti-inflammatory supplements daily for joint or other chronic pain, yet inflammation has benefits during the internal struggle to restore health. Reckeweg emphasizes the importance of this early inflammation phase in fighting disease, saying it is the mechanism by which the body cleanses and begins restoring or maintaining health. He charted six clinical stages of defense by the body.

Reckeweg's Six Clinical Stages of The Body's Defense

1) Phase-excretion, where toxins do not come in contact with epithelial cells but are absorbed and expelled with physiological secretions.
2) Phase-inflammation/reaction. Through the process of inflammation, the body neutralizes toxins and ejects them, yet some enter the flow system.

3) Phase-storage. Storage is followed by deactivation of the toxins in connective and fat tissue and in the vascular system.

4) Phase-impregnation. Here toxins are no longer localized but channeled into the distinguishing cells of a gland or organ and begin to dismantle the cell, attacking first its enzymatic mechanisms, with unfavorable prognoses.

5) Phase-degeneration. The continued accumulation of toxin saturation determines, after partial enzymatic block, the damage of intracellular organs and degeneration of tissues.

6) Phase-dedifferentiation. Chronic inflammatory stimulation of the cell can result in its differentiation into abnormal cells that, along with simultaneous weakening of the body's defenses, will take over the entire body.

An article by Dmitry Mednis, of the Medical Centre Bonamed in Kiev, Ukraine, discusses how today's doctors are over treating the early stages of disease and unwittingly contributing to a steady global increase in chronic illnesses. Mednis agrees with Reckeweg, saying "crisis" is a natural stage of the disease process. The problem is, there are a wide variety of treatment methods now available. If too much treatment is utilized during the early stages, the health challenge is kept at a low level and the body's "adaptive system" fails to consider it a significant threat. Mednis says allowing a disease to reach its natural crisis stage before treatment will result in the adaptive system mounting a stronger attack, instead of allowing low, chronic conditions to continue. He suggests biomedicine practitioners be trained to carefully monitor the body's own healing stages to avoid over treatment in early stages (April 2017, KeAi Publishing).

Resources:

Sheila Ring Reed, BioEnergetic Medicine & Homotoxicology, 12 Old Boston Post Road, Old Saybrook, CT 06475, www.sheilareed.net, Tel 860 577-0419

CHAPTER 3

BIORESONANCE THERAPY FOR DETOXIFICATION AND TREATMENT

According to quantum physics, all matter shares characteristics of being both waves and particles. Every living and non-living thing on earth emits electromagnetic waves and has its own frequency. This geomagnetic field rises from the Earth's core and extends roughly 600 miles into space. There it meets the solar wind, a stream of particles from the sun that recharge the Earth's frequency through lightning strikes. Thousands of lightning storms occur each day globally, with an estimated 1.4 billion flashes per year contributing to this planet's electromagnetic field.

Schumann Waves are quasi-standing electromagnetic waves having a very low frequency of 7.83 Hz, the same vibrational frequencies of our heart and brain. These waves exist between the Earth's surface and the ionosphere, a layer of the atmosphere that conducts electricity. Many experts believe the world-wide spectrum of artificial, man-made electromagnetic frequency (EMF) radiation in use today is masking the natural beneficial frequency of Earth, and this electropollution is causing its occupants to feel more stressed, fatigued, and unbalanced.

All cells in the body—as well as viruses, bacteria, pollen, and toxins—emit electromagnetic vibrations. Each microorganism has a unique frequency, as does each organ in the body. For example, healthy lungs resonate at a frequency around 72 Hertz, but when infected or impaired, the frequency drops. If the frequency of a healthy lung is reproduced using a frequency generator (discussed below), and that exact frequency is sent back into the body, the infected lung is strengthened by this additional energy and returns to its normal frequency and health.

For eradicating microorganisms and parasites, the principles of bioresonance still apply with one exception. When unhealthy frequencies are copied by a bioresonance device, they are "inverted" using an electronic circuit before being sent back into the body of the parasite. As soon as the altered frequency is absorbed by the organism, it ruptures and dies (see video in Resources). This is how unhealthy frequencies are deactivated in the body and healthy frequencies are supported. Bioresonance devices do not cure an illness. They simply assist the body by reducing its toxin and stress load, restoring its built-in "self-regulation."

BICOM Bioresonance Devices

There are several brands of bioresonance devices available, so I have chosen to discuss two companies. One is BICOM, the largest German provider of bioresonance devices for medical practitioners. The other is DETA-ELIS, a Russian company founded by a brother and sister who were involved in inventing bioresonance to keep Russian cosmonauts healthy while living on Russia's space station.

BICOM was started in the 1970s by Dr. Franz Morell, a German medical doctor who used Homeopathy in his practice. During that era, one of the leading theories on how Homeopathic remedies worked was that the water by which they were diluted and potentized somehow retained "memory" of its active ingredient. Since the human body is 70% water, if this theory was correct, Morell believed the "disease information" should somehow be stored in the water as well. He wondered if it might be possible to develop an "electronic Homeopathy" by using electromagnetic signals of the "disease" taken from the patient's body.

Joined by his electronic engineer son-in-law, Erich Rasche, the pair began working to create such a device. In 1977, bio-physicist Dr. Ludger Mersmann helped develop a filter to separate diseased electromagnetic signals in the body from healthy signals. The result was a biofeedback therapy device called the MORA. It used electrodes on the skin to pick up energetic signals throughout the body, modify them, and send them back into the patient to support healthy frequencies and cancel those causing diseases. The only drawback was it required time-consuming, manual set up.

Morell's colleague, Hans Brugeann, founded his own company (now Regumed GMbH) in 1987 and used a built-in computer to automate the operation. Regumed went on to make many technical improvements to the early BICOM device, including some in collaboration with other biophysics researchers. Today, BICOM offers a variety of models, with prices up to $26,000. Most are purchased by therapists for treating patients at fees ranging from $80 to $150 per hour.

There are now over 17,000 BICOM devices in use by medical practitioners and natural therapists in 80 countries. (The BICOM UK website is especially informative: https://bioresonance.com/introduction.) Widely known in Europe, bioresonance is gaining recognition as a complementary therapy in the US, Australia, and China, where BICOM devices are purchased by government hospitals for treating children.

Bioresonance Treats Many Conditions Contributing to Mental Disorders:

Addictions
Asthma
Allergies
Auto-immune disease
Dental infections
Electronic smog
Gastrointestinal diseases
Gynecological diseases
Headaches/migraines
Heavy metal toxicity
Hormone disorders
Inflammatory diseases
Lyme disease
Nervous system diseases
Parasites

Respiratory diseases
Skin diseases

DETA-ELIS Bioresonance Devices

The Russians developed a version of bioresonance therapy to meet the needs of cosmonauts living on the space station in the 1990s. All water on the station had to be filtered for reuse, so drugs and medications could not be taken by its residents. Dr. Sergei Konopliov and his sister, Tatiana Konopliova, worked with a group of experts and scientists for years to develop bioresonance devices and hold over 70 worldwide patents. In 1992, DETA-ELIS was founded by the pair in Zelenograd, Russia. It moved to Fulda, Germany (where the small devices are manufactured) in 2014 and became DETA-ELIS HOLDING, with the goal of selling its products globally.

Since I do not speak Russian, I became aware of DETA-ELIS through the website of Dr. George J. Georgiou, PhD, ND, DSc, (AM), a holistic medicine practitioner, researcher, author, and Director/Founder of Da Vinci Holistic Health Center (in Cyprus). Dr. Georgiou is also a brilliant and entertaining advocate. Plan to spend an hour or two learning and laughing when you visit his site www.deta-elis-uk.com. If you become serious about deepening your knowledge of bioresonance use, sign up for his online certification courses at the Da Vinci College of Holistic Medicine.

Why Dr. Georgiou chooses DETA-ELIS devices:

- An easy, efficient way to get rid of diseases without using drugs
- Helps many "incurable diseases," such as herpes, hepatitis C, tuberculosis, and others
- Can eliminate a wide variety of parasites not yet officially identified
- Safe to use with children and pets
- Is a highly efficient treatment method with no major side effects
- DETA ELIS offers 1600 treatment programs, having an overall positive effect of 85%.

DETA-ELIS Products Online

DETA-ELIS offers both professional treatment devices for practitioners and small, portable, wireless devices for consumers. Here is a sampling of those offered on-line.

The DETA PROFESSIONAL is created for medical practitioners and recognized by the Russian Ministry of Health, Israel, and other countries as an official method of diagnosis. Its Diagnostic Mode uses bioresonance testing to check for parasites, bacteria, fungi, viruses, organ imbalances, underlying causes of diseases, drug interactions in the patient, scar, sinus, tooth and tonsil foci, food intolerances, and imbalances in meridians and chakras.

In Therapy Mode, the DETA PROFESSIONAL is capable of delivering five different methods of treatment: electro-acupuncture, electromagnetic therapy, quantum healing, bioresonance therapy, or a combination of these. Sold to qualified health practitioners, it requires extensive training to use. The listed price in Euros is €7,950. At the November 2017 Euro/Dollar currency exchange rate of $1.18 for €1.00, the US price would be $9,381.

The DEVITA RITM 30 is an in-home device for personal or family use, designed for upregulating organ systems in the body. Over 1,650 separate frequencies can be utilized to restore normal functioning of organs and systems, quietly and painlessly with resonant frequencies. At the same time, the device can be used for detoxifying. It was shown beneficial in many Russian studies for treating cardiovascular problems, endocrine disorders, urological diseases, gastrointestinal problems, headaches, inflammatory conditions, respiratory system malfunctions, and central and peripheral nervous system diseases. The on-line price for the DEVITA RITM 30, using the November 2017 Euro/Dollar exchange given above, is €599, or $707. Manufactured in Germany, it has CE certification as an Electromagnetic Wellness Device.

The DEVITA AP 30 is a new model that comes with 30 pre-installed programs and is mainly used for eradicating parasites, bacteria, fungi, viruses and many other disease-causing microorganisms. A partial list of new programs added include: anti-cold frequencies, anti-flu, anti-virus, digestive tract help, two drainage programs for toxic accumulation, a program for genitourinary infections, no allergies, no bacteria, no chlamydia, no fungi, no helicobacter, no hepatitis A, no hepatitis B, and four no herpes programs (with others listed on line).

The AP 30 also contains specific frequencies for 90 different types of viruses, 91 types of bacteria, 61 types of fungi, 31 types of protozoa, and 33 types of helminths. Further frequencies are included to eliminate roundworms, *Mycoplasma, Trichomoniasis,* onychomycosis, *Staphylococcus, Streptococcus, Chlamydia,* herpes virus, Epstein-Barr virus, cytomegalovirus, *Candida,* and others (listed on line).

By matching the frequency or vibration exactly, any microorganisms will absorb the inverted energy, burst, and die. Programs can be run for 30-40 days, but any microbe treatment should always be followed by running a drainage program to clear debris from the body. The DEVITA AP 30 is listed at €599, or $707. Manufactured in Germany, it has a CE certification as an Electromagnetic Wellness Device and received numerous awards and medals from scientific organizations for its achievements in advancing wellness.

During its 20 years of research and development, DETA-ELIS has conducted 120 clinical studies. A few research summaries conducted between 1995 and 2010 have been translated from Russian and are available at http://www.deta-elis-uk.com/clinical-studies.

All three healing methods discussed in Part I of this book—Homeopathy, Homotoxicology, and BioResonance Therapy—were soundly rejected by conventionally trained, Western medical practitioners before high powered electron microscopes, advances in quantum physics, and massive use of the treatments by poor countries revealed one thing: these therapies consistently help patients.

Resources

Regumed GMbH official web site: https://www.regumed.com

BICOM UK web site: https://bioresonance.com/introduction

BICOM UK Kick Smoking Video: https://bioresonance.com/smoking

BICOM UK Lyme Disease info: https://bioresonance.com/disorders/lyme

BICOM UK Scientific Papers: https://bioresonance.com/scientific-papers

DETA-ELIS official website: http://deholding.gr/us

DETA-ELIS video: DEVITA AP 30 device frequency killing parasite:

http://www.deta-elis-uk.com/deta-ap

DETA-ELIS UK: www.deta-elis-uk.com

DETA-ELIS clinical studies http://www.deta-elis-uk.com/clinical-studies

PART II
REBALANCING THE BRAIN

CHAPTER 4

FISHER WALLACE STIMULATOR FOR DEPRESSION, ANXIETY, INSOMNIA, AND PAIN

Medical engineer Saul Liss and his brother Bernard obtained patent No. 5,109,847 for what was considered a "TENS" device (transcutaneous electrical nerve stimulator) in 1990. The device went through several variations before being called the Liss Cranial Electrical Stimulator. In May 1992, *The New York Times* reported that Dr. C. Norman Shealy, a well-known neurosurgeon, had used the Liss device at Shealy Institute for Comprehensive Pain for years.

On September 11, 2001, when the Twin Towers were attacked in New York City, the late Dr. Martin Wallace, PhD, CCN, CAd, was trapped for eight hours in a building at Ground Zero. Following the attack, he developed acute depression and was unable to find successful treatment. Wallace joined forces with Charles ("Chip") Avery Fisher, the son of stereo pioneer Avery Fisher, and the partners discovered a poorly-marketed, yet effective FDA sanctioned medical device—the LISS Cranial Stimulator—that rapidly relieved Wallace's depression without causing any side effects. They purchased all of its patents from Dr. Saul Liss and co-founded Fisher Wallace Labs in 2006, with Fisher serving as President.

In 2014, the Fisher Wallace Stimulator (FWS) was approved for use by all 11 hospitals in the New York City Health and Hospitals Corporation, including Bellevue, Woodhull, Jacobi, Kings County, Metropolitan, Lincoln, Queens, and North Central Bronx hospitals. Dr. Richard Brown, Associate Clinical Professor of Psychiatry, and colleagues at Columbia University have documented prescribing the FWS to over 750 patients for treatment of depression, anxiety, and insomnia, with a 70% effectiveness rate—roughly twice that of antidepressants!

By 2016, Forbes magazine called the Fisher Wallace Stimulator "one of four technologies innovating mental health," citing its safety and effectiveness shown by 11 published studies. The Fisher Wallace Stimulator has been prescribed by over 6,000 providers and now sells over 10,000 devices a year.

Fisher Wallace Stimulator

The Fisher Wallace Stimulator is a cranial electrotherapy device approved by the FDA for treatment of depression, anxiety, insomnia, and chronic pain. The portable, hand-held system uses micro-electrical currents with patented frequencies to stimulate the brain's production of "feel-good" neurotransmitters serotonin, dopamine, and GABA, along with Beta-endorphin and DHEA hormones.

At the same time, Fisher Wallace frequencies lower levels of cortisol, a stress hormone that, when chronically high, hinders one's ability to sleep. In children, high cortisol levels damage the developing brain, resulting in less white matter (used for communications). Too much cortisol also stunts collection and recall of new information, which impairs a child's ability to learn, lowering IQ by as much as 10 points in some studies.

For treatment, two moistened sponge electrodes are held in place on the temples with a headband. (In cases of chronic or acute pain, electrodes are applied to the body rather than the temples.) The device is activated by turning a small wheel, which shuts off automatically after 20 minutes. Powered by AA batteries, it is safe to use with or without medications and presents no safety concerns.

Additional Uses

Two recent studies have examined additional uses for the Fisher Wallace Stimulator. A proof-of-concept, functional MRI (fMRI) study was undertaken in 2011 to develop an innovative method for obtaining fMRI resting-state network maps during electrical stimulation of the brain (ESB). The concept was that non-invasive ESB modifies the resting-state network connectivity of the primary motor cortex. The stimulation appears to undo some deficits in neural network communication and improve connectivity within the central nervous system. This type of study will help understand more of the mechanisms responsible for therapeutic benefits from non-invasive ESB. But to do the study, an innovative method for obtaining fMRI resting-state network maps during electrical stimulation had to be developed and tested.

Five healthy volunteers participated in two fMRI sessions. The first session used a transcranial direct current stimulator, while the second used the Fisher Wallace monophasic pulsed current stimulator. The human fMRI data clearly indicated that measurable changes occurred in left primary motor cortex brain tissue directly under the stimulating electrode. Researchers concluded both devices can safely be applied within a 3 T magnet without any signal degradation. Further, non-invasive electric stimulation of the brain provides a calming effect by lowering cortisol and turning off the state of vigilance in anxious patients. Stimulation effects are persistent for at least 13 minutes post-stimulation, and the magnitude of resting-state change may or may not depend on which type of electrical stimulation is used (Alon G, et al. Brain Res, 2011).

Bipolar patients spend three times as many days depressed as hypomanic or manic patients. A 2015 double-blind, sham-controlled study was conducted of patients experiencing Bipolar II Depression who received daily treatment with the Fisher Wallace Stimulator for 20 minutes five days a week for two weeks. The sham group's device was turned on for 20 minutes but did not deliver any micro-electrical currents, then it automatically turned off. Neither group knew who had received the real treatment. Both groups received an additional two weeks of open-label active treatment. Researchers found a significant decrease in the Beck Depression Inventory scores from baseline to the second week, which were maintained until the study ended after four weeks. The device was shown to be a safe and effective treatment for Bipolar II Depression (McClure, et al, Jr Nervous and Mental Disease, 2015). Its low cost, portability, and lack of side effects make it especially appealing to patients.

There is also some evidence that the FWS may provide treatment for veterans suffering from the effects of brutality and war. US Marine Corps veteran Logan Shield describes how the Fisher Wallace device helped him recover mental stability following four tours of duty in six years and multiple suicide attempts, the first at age 12 during a childhood filled with anxiety and depression: https://www.fisherwallace.com/pages/patient-doctor-testimonials.

Later in the same video, retired US Army Brigadier General Stephen Xenakis, MD, a psychiatrist with 20-years of active duty, says many soldiers experience multiple problems. The most common one is difficulty sleeping. "This device helps with sleep, anxiety, and mood, which helps thinking, attention, and concentration. We also have lots of evidence it (the device) does very little, if any, harm at all. I prescribe it as an adjunctive treatment.... Many patients have used it for years." Veterans may find the videos at www.FisherWallace.com helpful.

Cranial stimulation research has consistently shown improvement for substance abuse as well. A rehabilitation clinic, Phoenix House in New York City, revealed that use of the FWS increased its 90-day patient retention rates by 50% in a 392-patient pilot program. Earlier studies were published under a variety of descriptive names: Transcranial Electric Treatment (USSR), Neuroelectric Therapy (England), and Electrosleep (Texas).

Side Effects

Kids should never be prescribed drugs when safer treatment options exist. Psychiatric drugs interact with hormones and reduce a child's growth. Plus, they have a long list of side effects, which are not discussed with patients until after they occur. Side effects for antidepressants include dry mouth, drowsiness or insomnia, dizziness, diarrhea, constipation, headache, and weight gain of 30-60 pounds or loss of weight. Less frequent but more severe side effects are increased depression and suicidal tendencies; neurologically driven agitation, ranging from mild leg tapping to severe panic; tics or muscle spasms; and Parkinsonism. Prozac and Luvox are known to increase the risk of inducing mania in children. These are just a few of the reasons I was delighted to meet Chip Fisher and learn about this simple, effective, device that is so safe kids can use it at home.

In two National Institute of Health studies, SSRI antidepressants caused side effects in 38% of patients, yet prove effective in only 31% of patients within 14 weeks. The Fisher Wallace Stimulator causes only minor side effects in less than 1% of patients. Published studies show it is effective in over

60% of patients overall, and in more than 70% of patients from large clinical practices.

The FWS Kit retails for $699 and includes everything needed for use:

- Fisher Wallace Stimulator
- Headset
- White Velcro Headband
- (6) Sponges
- AA batteries
- White Velcro Body Strap (for pain treatment)
- Carrying case
- Insomnia, Anxiety, Depression instruction manual
- Chronic Pain instruction manual

Made in the USA, it comes with a one-year warranty. The company also has a 30-day return and refund policy.

Many but not all private insurance companies, such as Aetna, United Healthcare and Blue Cross have reimbursed patients for the purchase of the Fisher Wallace Stimulator, especially when it is used for the treatment of pain. The company does not process reimbursement claims on behalf of patients. It recommends contacting your insurance provider to confirm coverage and learn how to obtain reimbursement. A health care authorization from any licensed practitioner is required for coverage. The Fisher Wallace web site offers a free template of the Purchase Authorization Form for download, along with additional information on the reimbursement process.

Kortex - A Neurostimulating VR Headset

In 2017, Fisher Wallace introduced Kortex—the world's first neurostimulation device designed for Virtual Reality (VR) headsets—led by Kelly Roman, Co-Founder and VR strategy leader. Kortex utilizes the same proprietary technology as the Fisher Wallace Stimulator and is the company's first wearable device. Both stimulate the brain to produce serotonin, a feel-good neurotransmitter, along with the sleep hormone, melatonin, while lowering the stress hormone, cortisol.

Launched on crowdfunding site Indiegogo, Kortex exceeded its fundraising goal within two weeks. The device was shipped to customers in November 2017 and will have its own site once the Indigogo campaign version is completed. Until then, it is only available at https://www.indiegogo.com/search#/?q=Kortex.

Kortex easily attaches to most VR headsets, including the Samsung Gear VR, Google Daydream, and ZEISS VR ONE Plus. The company has partnered with usTwo Games (makers of Monument Valley) to provide every Kortex user a free copy of their award-winning Land's End VR game. Many other VR experiences, such as Relax VR, are freely downloadable.

Engaging virtual reality content helps improve the user experience and compliance. Virtual reality therapy is also used to treat PTSD as well as substance abuse recovery patients and others. Prescription VR therapy may be amplified by use of Kortex.

Unlike the Fisher Wallace Stimulator, which is FDA regulated, Kortex is classified as a general wellness device and intended to help manage sleep and stress. As a result, it may be obtained without a prescription. Best results come from using Kortex once or twice a day for 20 minutes. Most people will notice results during the first two weeks of daily use.

Resources:

Fisher Wallace Laboratories, 515 Madison Ave, 22nd Floor, New York, NY 10022, Tel 212 688-8100, www.fisherwallace.com

Kortex on Indiegogo: https://www.indiegogo.com/search#/?q=Kortex

CHAPTER 5

BRAIN BALANCE ACHIEVEMENT CENTERS FOR ADHD, AUTISM, DYSLEXIA, TOURETTE'S

In the early 1990s, Dr. Robert Melillo, a chiropractic neurologist, professor, and researcher, noticed an increase in the number of children coming to his practice with learning and behavioral issues. He began a passionate search for a clearer understanding of ADHD, Dyslexia, Processing Disorders, and Autism Spectrum Disorders. Through his research and extensive clinical experience, he came to consider these disorders as indicators of an underlying problem in the brain, called Functional Disconnection Syndrome. This imbalance in brain development was the common thread among the learning and behavioral issues.

A brain normally communicates between both hemispheres at lightning speed. When communications between the right and left hemispheres are abnormal, often due to not maturing at the same rate, the underdeveloped side runs at a slower speed. Without sufficient neuronal connections and a compatible processing speed, children become partially disconnected from their bodies and senses. This, in turn, causes behavioral, emotional, social, and learning difficulties. Most developmental issues, however, can be avoided or corrected if treated early in life.

Dr. Melillo began implementing his integrated approach to helping children in 1994. He spent 12 years refining the program—a non-medical, non-pharmaceutical approach that does not rely on drugs, medical procedures, or psychotherapy. The results were positive and compelling, demonstrating the program's success at correcting a fundamental imbalance between the two hemispheres of the brain by integrating the three pillars of brain development in its protocol: sensory motor stimulation, cognitive stimulation, and nutrition.

Brain Balance is the only method I am aware of that treats the many dysfunctions of developmental imbalance concurrently in one customized 12 to 36-week program. For most parents, it is a relief to work with just one practitioner weekly, instead of several. Plus, this innovative treatment often restores a child's ability to function normally, avoiding a variety of life-long therapies with overwhelming costs. The results can be dramatic, in one case even transforming a child who had never spoken before into a happy, social, academic achiever.

A Child Speaks for First Time in 8 Years

"What a great program and the staff is WONDERFUL. When we started this program, I was skeptical. When I originally met with Dr. Pete he gave me some home exercises to do and I started them that night. THE NEXT morning for the first time in 8 years, my child said good morning to me! I was like what? Evidently, we stimulated something in the brain to make her more aware. Since then, the changes have been great. She can speak in full sentences, can focus better at school and is more aware of her surroundings. I have another child that also has gone through this program and the changes in her are significant! Next year, she will no longer need adaptive PE, Occupational Therapy, or a Parapro to assist in specials! Our pediatrician is amazed with the differences in my children, as are all of our friends and family...." Eileen H.

Treatment

The Brain Balance Achievement Centers treat ADHD, Asperger's Syndrome, High Functioning Autism, Pervasive Developmental Disorder, Dyslexia, Tourette's Syndrome, processing disorders, and other spectrum disorders

Creating an individualized treatment plan begins with a comprehensive assessment performed at one of the centers. A child's functioning ability is tested in three areas: 1) sensorimotor, 2) neuro-academic, and 3) bio-nutritional. The assessment includes over 200 individual measurements in sensory-motor, vestibular, auditory, vision proprioception (knowing where one's body is in space), tactile, and olfactory skills.

A customized 12-week treatment program includes therapy to improve balance and communication between the brain's two hemispheres, given for one hour, three times a week. Sensory, motor and cognitive work are used to strengthen weak brain areas, pushing them to catch up, grow new connections, increase processing speed, and establish a normal, balanced rhythm.

Academic activities target improving specific academic skills and subjects, to stimulate growth and development in the part of the brain controlling that skill. The goal is to help each child get back on track academically in:

- Word reading
- Reading comprehension
- Pseudo-decoding
- Math reasoning
- Numerical operations
- Listening comprehension
- Oral expression
- Spelling
- Written expression

Nutritional guidance is used to address the root cause of many neurobehavioral issues. Gluten intolerance and other undiagnosed food sensitivities often contribute to mental dysfunction. Environmental toxins (mercury, lead, pesticides, PCBs, etc.) are notorious contributors as well. Family education during treatment includes a dietary program with supplements for each child aimed at correcting nutrient deficiencies and optimizing brain function. At-home exercises complement the work done in the center, with its frequency and duration contributing to each child's progress.

Successful treatment is typically measured by "normal" and age-appropriate behavior and achievement. According to an independent control study among students who participated in the Brain Balance program, published in the peer reviewed *Frontiers in Child Health and Human Development:*

- 81% of children who completed the program no longer met the criteria for ADHD, based on standardized behavioral testing.
- approximately 60% of children studied showed a minimum of a two-grade level increase in a variety of academic testing. An additional 35% of these children showed a four-grade increase or better, based on academic achievement testing after 12 weeks.
- 100% of children in the study showed some improvement in more than one area including: listening skills, spelling skills, mathematic reasoning, reading comprehension, written and oral abilities.

The Brain Balance program is offered to families on a private-pay basis. Total cost is determined by how many weeks are needed to achieve the desired results. The initial assessment cost is $295 for each child. Most programs range from 12 to 36 weeks, with a 12-week program priced at $6,500, including all lab work. Dietary supplements range from $100 to $150 for the three-month period.

"My child before Brain Balance

Ryan had ADHD, Tourette's and OCD. He was not able to complete daily tasks because his ADHD was so severe. His tics were so bad that they would keep him up at night, and some would cause pain and repetitive injury. Ryan's OCD was so bad that he could not complete his homework due to his hand writing never being "perfect." He was emotionally volatile and prone to outbursts. He was on five different brain-chemical altering medications, none of which helped.

"My child after Brain Balance

Ryan gets up every morning and gets dressed and brushes his teeth without having to be reminded. He is consistently getting all stars on his progress reports at school and he completes his homework every night with no issues. His anger outbursts are gone. He is happy, attentive, and follows directions without prompts or reminders. He is more outgoing, calm, and has more self-esteem. He still has some small tics. However, they are nowhere near where they used to be. He has been taken off all of his meds due to his profound improvement! Ryan also received student of the year award at his school!"

--Victoria B.

A "Hot" Wellness Franchise

Aware there were thousands of families desperately seeking hope and tangible help, Dr. Melillo was determined to make the Brain Balance approach available to as many children as possible. Under the direction of William Fowler, Dr. Melillo's business partner and a pioneer in business development, Brain Balance Center Franchises were offered for sale in 2006. Franchising enabled rapid, precise replication. In 2013, *CNN Money* named Brain Balance one of the "5 Hot Franchises."

A 2013 profile of Fowler in *Entrepreneur Magazine* named the Brain Balance franchise one of six start-up-friendly industries that is "booming despite the gloomy economy."

A development team supports new franchisees' selection of a location, architect, and contractors. Normally located in a busy, upscale strip mall with plenty of parking, Brain Balance Centers include large, airy play and exercise space, designed to welcome kids of all ages, along with offices and meeting rooms.

Proprietary Brain Balance software provides oversight and management of the center from anywhere in the world at any time. A sophisticated business model helps owners leverage their capital, labor, and marketing as they open and manage one or multiple centers. Experienced Brain Balance staff are available for hands-on-training and consulting. Soon owners are able to deliver daily student program activities and reports to parents in real time. The system's tremendous data collection capability also supports on-going research, increases in efficiency and productivity, as well as franchise growth.

Brain Balance Centers continue to expand rapidly, with 100 currently operating in the United States and 30 more under development. For parents and others interested in a profitable investment that will also make a pivotal difference in children's lives, telephone (866) 344-6600, or go to franchise. brainbalancecenters.com.

Research

To assist patients and parents, Dr. Melillo has authored several books: *Neurobehavioral Disorders of Childhood* (2004), a working theory textbook on developmental disabilities; his best-selling book, *Disconnected Kids* (2009); *Reconnected Kids* (2011); and *Autism - The Scientific Truth About Preventing, Diagnosing and Treating Autism Spectrum Disorders* (2012). His most recent release is *The Disconnected Kids Nutrition Plan.*

Melillo has also published numerous scientific papers and contributed chapters to 10 professional books that support Brain Balance Centers' methods.

If you are intrigued by this unique approach, here is a link to a 2009 paper written by Drs. Melillo and Gerry Leisman (*Rev Neuroscience*, 20(2):111-31), outlining how a functional disconnection would explain all of the symptoms of autistic spectrum disorder: http://drrobertmelillo.com/research/2009-Melillo-Leisman-Autism-RevNeuro-rev220509.pdf.

Resources:

Brain Balance Website: https://www.brainbalancecenters.com/, Tel 1-800 877 5500

Brain Balance Overview, 10 min: https://www.youtube.com/watch?v=AvDQ 8m9DZzQ

Brain Balance in action video: https://www.youtube.com/watch?v=vqXPzv H4nfs

Brain Balance Franchise info: franchise.brainbalancecenters.com, Tel 866 344-6600

Dr. Melillo, 20 videos: https://www.youtube.com/user/drrobertmelillo

Weiler 9-yr-old son Testimonial: https://www.youtube.com/watch?v=8Zu7Ui-wefY

CHAPTER 6

NuCalm For Stress, Insomnia, and Pain

A great deal of research indicates today's fast-paced, over-scheduled family lives are directly fueling the epidemics of childhood stress, insomnia, obesity, and mental illness. This chapter will explain how all these ailments are connected, like segments of a dragon. What parents and kids can do to eliminate this beast is chop off its head – STRESS. NuCalm, makes it easy.

In 2002, Solace Lifesciences, Inc., began creating a treatment to help people lower stress and improve sleep quality without drugs. After eight years of research and development, NuCalm was launched in 2010 by the pioneering neuroscientist and Solace Founder, Dr. G. Blake Holloway. Its patented, all natural, scientifically sequenced system uses the body's own communication pathways to interrupt the stress response, quickly guiding brain waves into a deeply relaxed state.

A session begins by applying a topical cream, or chewing a proprietary blend of dietary supplements, that contains the natural amino acid Gamma-Aminobutyric Acid (known as GABA), to prepare the brain for relaxation. Another ingredient, L-Theanine, is an amino acid found in tea plants that supports formation of GABA as well as contributes to feelings of calm and well-being.

After being seated in a reclining lounge chair, neuro-patches are applied directly behind both ears to enable cranial electrotherapy stimulation—a subsensory microcurrent to help catalyze the effects of the supplements and accelerate the relaxation response. The microcurrent presents an electrical signal that is close to the cell's own electrical values, to help the brain's neurochemistry by reestablishing optimal neurotransmitter levels.

Headphones are used to provide proprietary neuro-acoustic software that brings the pace of brain waves to pre-sleep levels of 12Hz -4Hz. A light-blocking eye mask helps prevent visual stimulation and maintain the deeply relaxed state for the entire treatment. NuCalm treatments typically last between 20-40 minutes, based on what a person is experiencing—the more stress, the longer the treatment. NuCalm improves sleep quality for most clients, along with mood, focus, decision making, productivity, immune function, and health.

Recently, a close friend mentioned she had been unable to sleep soundly for months due to extreme back pain at night. She accompanied me to the office of Chris Deveau, DC, who upon hearing about her pain offered an introductory NuCalm session for relief. It did something even more surprising. In less than five minutes, my friend was sound asleep in the recliner, and remained so during the entire session. When a soft chime indicated her time was up, she awoke astonished, exclaiming she had not slept that well or felt so good in weeks!

Professional athletes were quick to embrace NuCalm. Their list of routine stressors is long: dieting and sleep issues, perpetual travel, off-season training, regular and post season games, overtraining, injuries, recuperation, contract negotiations, and juggling to meet family, sponsor, and social obligations.

According to coaches and trainers, making NuCalm part of an athlete's ritual helps them sleep better, recover more fully from injuries, and deliver peak performance in decisive moments. Deep relaxation clears their mind of distractions and helps remove self-doubt. Not surprisingly, NuCalm is currently used by athletes in the NFL, NHL, MLB, and NBA.

Chronic Stress and Insomnia

When faced with frightening physical or emotional challenges, the body automatically releases a cascade of stress hormones known as the "fight-or-flight" response. Directed by the autonomic nervous system that controls other involuntary body functions, this vast network of nerves reaches from the spinal cord to all organs. Its two main branches have opposite effects. The first branch, our sympathetic nervous system, releases stress hormones the instant our brain perceives a threat.

We all recognize the familiar adrenaline "rush." Our heart rate and breathing speed up, carrying energy and oxygen to cells, elevating blood pressure, and narrowing our focus, as our muscles tense, preparing for escape. Adrenaline is assisted by norepinephrine, which makes you alert, quick to act. It also shifts blood flow to crucial parts of the body to release glucose (blood sugar) from energy stores, increasing blood flow to skeletal muscles and lowering its flow to the intestines. Adrenaline causes arteries to narrow, pumping blood harder and faster to assist escape.

Cortisol—a steroid acting like a stress hormone—also joins the rush during fight-or-flight. In a crisis, it floods the body with glucose to energize large muscles and the brain, enhancing memory and elevating your pain threshold. Cortisol also temporarily inhibits production of insulin to prevent blood sugar from being stored, keeping it available for immediate use. Plus, it temporarily down-regulates digestion, the immune system, and other non-essential activity during a crisis.

Once the threat has passed, the parasympathetic branch of the autonomic nervous system takes over to restore normal balance. Cortisol levels begin to drop. Insulin is no longer inhibited by too much cortisol and it resumes controlling blood sugar levels. We calm down and relax, with no short-term ill effects.

Daily chronic stress, however, prevents this return to normal and is responsible for the "adult" health problems now occurring in kids. It is especially damaging when brains are developing because it impairs the ability to learn. In England, a study of 1,116 five-year-old twin pairs found children who experienced high levels of domestic violence had IQs averaging eight points lower than those not exposed (Koenen KC, et al, 2003). Other studies of kids experiencing verbal abuse, domestic violence, or "household chaos" reported lower IQs, lower reading achievement by almost ten points, and more conduct problems.

In Israel, Germany, the USA, China, and Italy, lab rats were given daily injections of rat cortisol for several weeks. It killed brain cells in the hippocampus area, where information is transferred from short-term memory into long-term memory, thus stunting their ability to retain new information. The rodents became depressed, anxious, fearful, immature, needy, and unable to learn new behaviors.

After a stressed-out day, excess cortisol lingers in the system, hindering sleep. Odd as it may seem, the longer you go without sleep the harder it is to get to sleep, because sleep deprivation also elevates cortisol. Many people shrug, saying, "I've lived on a few hours of sleep all my life. My body is used to it." But short sleep dramatically increases the risk of serious health challenges, including high blood pressure, diabetes, obesity, heart attack, stroke, and accelerated aging.

Sleep is not a luxury. It is an essential that delivers significant health benefits and prevents significant health problems. Why? *While you are sleeping—when other internal activities are at rest—the body makes cellular repairs and regeneration.* A 14-year study of insomnia found that those who experienced chronic insomnia (less than six hours of sleep a night) were four times more likely to die earlier in life than those with healthy sleep patterns (Vgontzas, 2010, *Sleep*).

Hours of Sleep Required to Maintain Health
New guidelines from the National Sleep Foundation

Newborns 0 to 3 months, **14 to 17 hours** of sleep every 24 hours (including naps)

Infants 4-12 months, **12 to 15 hours** of sleep every 24 hours (including naps)

Toddlers 1 to 2 years, **11 to 14 hours** of sleep every 24 hours (including naps)

Preschoolers 3 to 5 years, **10 to 13 hours** of sleep every 24 hours (including naps)

Children 6 to 13 years, **9 to 11 hours** of sleep every 24 hours

Teens 13 to 18 years, **8 to 10 hours** of sleep every 24 hours

Younger adults 18 to 25 years, **7 to 9 hours** of sleep every 24 hours

Adults 26 to 64 years, **7 to 9 hours** of sleep every 24 hours

Older adults 65+ years, **7 to 8 hours** of sleep every 24 hours

There are four stages of sleep that together make up one sleep cycle. The first three stages are when the body primarily performs cellular repairs and restoration. Each stage features non-rapid eye movement behind closed eyelids, referred to as NREM, NREM2, and NREM3 (the latter is also called slow-wave-sleep). Most dreaming occurs during rapid eye movement sleep (REM). In REM sleep, all muscles, except for the eyes' and those used to breathe, are temporarily paralyzed. REM sleep has more active brain wave patterns than

NREM stages, and scientists believe this part of the cycle is devoted exclusively to brain functions. Each complete cycle lasts 90-120 minutes and is repeated four to five times a night.

Sleep medications should not be given to children. They disturb both REM and non-REM sleep activity and can be habit-forming. Side effects from sleeping pills include sleepiness during the day, dizziness, lightheadedness, poor muscle coordination, and impaired mental functioning. Some kids sleep walk, eat, or even make phone calls under the effects of sleep medications, with no recollection of their actions. Sleep disruptions, like nightmares, chills, sweating, sleepwalking, restlessness, headache, trembling, confusion, anxiety, and irritability, are commonly caused by low blood sugar. Giving your child breakfast, lunch, dinner, plus two small snacks in between, helps keep blood sugar levels and moods more stable.

Safe, Natural Ways to Improve Sleep

Exercise 30-60 minutes, 3-4 times weekly, to produce "feel-good" endorphins.

Avoid caffeine after mid-day.

Reduce stress through meditation, muscle relaxation, or brain wave balancing.

Eat a light dinner to keep indigestion from interfering with sleep.

Go to bed and arise at the same time every day, "training" your body when to sleep.

Sleep the number of hours recommended for your age each night.

Sleep in loose fitting clothes.

Keep bedroom slightly cool.

Sleep in darkness, covering all LED lights.

Look at bright light first thing in the morning to help you wake up.

Remove TV and computers from the bedroom (even for adults).

Melatonin supplements, milk, the herbs Chamomile and Ashwagandha root enhance sleep.

Consult trained therapists to resolve sleep anxiety or worries.

Connecting Insomnia, Obesity, and Mental Health

Let's review the links involved. Chronic stress elevates cortisol and prevents restful sleep. Insomnia increases stress and triggers even more cortisol production. High cortisol temporarily inhibits insulin storage, thus flooding the body with insulin. Insulin is also known as "the hunger hormone," since high levels urge us to snack and result in slow but steady weight gain. To protect themselves, cells become insulin resistant, which over time brings the diagnosis of type II diabetes. This steady march toward obesity and diabetes is the direct result of excess cortisol from daily stress followed by too little sleep.

Or, it might be leptin's fault. Leptin hormones control thermogenesis, a process that helps burn fat. When leptin levels are low your metabolism slows down, and appetite is stimulated. After a meal, leptin levels rise, delivering a feeling of fullness, and speeding up metabolism. Certain lifestyle choices lead to "leptin resistance," where metabolism is not stimulated nor is appetite suppressed, making weight loss almost impossible. What are these lifestyle choices? Stress, fast food, insufficient exercise, and insufficient sleep.

Analysis of short-sleep and obesity studies—which included 634,511 children and adults from around the world, ages 2 to 102—consistently showed an increased risk of obesity among children and adults who were "short sleepers" (Cappuccio, et al, 2008). The review of 11 other studies in children ages 5-16 from Japan, Portugal, Germany, France, Canada, Brazil, Tunisia, Taiwan, Senegal, and United States, found short sleep duration "strongly and consistently associated with concurrent and future obesity" (Patel SR, Hu FB, *Obesity*, 2008).

A 2015 study, "Addressing Childhood Obesity: Opportunities for Prevention" (Brown CL, Appel, et al), offered a comprehensive list of kids' obesity risk factors:

- Genetics
- increased personal, prenatal, or family stress
- short sleep duration
- lower physical activity
- high intake of sugar-sweetened beverages, fast-food, and processed snacks (junk foods)
- environmental and neighborhood conditions

Sleep problems are so commonly found along with mental diagnoses they were once listed as symptoms in the psychiatric industry's *Diagnostic and Statistical Manual*. A study of 183 young children in an early childhood psychiatric day treatment program found 41% of children met the criteria for having a sleep disorder in addition to a mental disorder (Boekamp JR, et al, 2015).

Overweight children frequently experience anxiety and/or depression. A 2013 study at a pediatric obesity clinic examined cortisol profiles among 128 obese children, ages 2 to 11 years, and found symptoms of anxiety and/or depression associated with higher cortisol levels. Obese children were 3.5 times more likely to report anxiety and 3.6 times more likely to be depressed than controls (*Stress*, 2013).

Connections between insomnia, sleep movement, and mental health symptoms were examined in another 14-year study of 396 children. Patterns of insomnia and sleep-related movement from ages 4.5 to 9 years were considered, as well as associations with mental health symptoms in childhood, and long-term sleep problems that continued with mental health symptoms at ages 9 and 18. Researchers concluded such associations are common, and interestingly, that symptom persistence from middle to late childhood predicted specific types of mental health symptoms at age 18 (Armstrong JM, et al, Sleep 2014).

Reducing stress before it leads to insomnia, obesity and mental disorders is far easier than trying to reverse this process later. NuCalm is designed to interrupt living with chronic stress and reset the body's ability to fall into deep, rejuvenating sleep. Helping kids develop healthy sleep habits is a gift that will serve them into adolescence and adulthood. When a good night's sleep is combined with eating wholesome foods, daily exercise, and good lifestyle choices, your child will have the keys to maintaining health throughout their life.

Resources:

NuCalm: Solace Lifesciences, Inc., 501 Silverside Rd, #7, Wilmington, DE 19809, Tel 877 668-2256, www.nucalm.com

CHAPTER 7

NEUROFEEDBACK BRAIN TRAINING FOR MOST MENTAL DIAGNOSES

Biofeedback is a field of science that has been successful at teaching patients to consciously regulate autonomic body functions, such as heart rate and blood pressure, and to regulate damaged muscles. An outgrowth of biofeedback, neurofeedback ("neuro" referring to the nervous system) was developed in the 1960s by several groups of researchers. It became the fastest-growing area of biofeedback, using electroencephalograms (EEGs) to measure brain-wave activity and train patients to deliberately change this activity.

The father of contemporary neurofeedback is Professor Emeritus Barry Sterman of the University of California's Los Angeles School of Medicine. He discovered that laboratory cats, when trained through operant conditioning, could increase a certain range of brain waves and greatly elevate their resistance to developing seizure activity. This led Sterman to help patients having chronic seizures and poor medication responses become seizure free. He and his students continued refining these techniques for treatment of ADHD, brain injuries, anxiety, depression and other mental disorders. Today brain-wave training is called EEG biofeedback or neurofeedback.

Brainwaves

Brainwaves have various frequencies, from very fast to extremely slow. The classical names of these EEG band widths are Delta, Theta, Alpha, Beta, and Gamma. Their frequencies are measured in cycles per second, or hertz (Hz). Brainwaves appear to play a major role in brain timing and network function.

Brainwave Frequency Ranges:

- Delta waves (.5 to 3 Hz) are very slow, loud brainwaves, of low frequency that indicate a deep, restorative sleep
- Theta waves (3 to 8 Hz) are associate with light, healthy sleep, frequencies important in infancy childhood, and young adults
- Alpha waves (8 to 12 Hz) are indicative of relaxed wakefulness and meditative states; in lower ranges, the brain appears to be idling, a bit disengaged
- Beta waves (12 to 38 Hz) occur when fully awake, with eyes open and an outward-focused concentration on intellectual activity
- Gamma waves (38 to 42 Hz), are very fast and believed to indicate intensely focused intention and to help process and bind together information from other areas of the brain (Hammond D, *Jr Neurotherapy*, 2011)

We all have some degree of these frequencies present in different parts of our brain. For instance, if someone is very anxious and tense, the high frequency of beta brainwaves may be present in several places. People with ADD, ADHD, head injury, stroke, epilepsy, chronic fatigue, fibromyalgia, or developmental disabilities often have excess slow theta and alpha waves present in several places. When too many slow waves are in the frontal lobes where executive functioning occurs, that person will struggle with concentration, memory, controlling impulses and moods, and exhibit diminished intellect (Hammond D, *Jr Neurotherapy*, 2011).

Brain Training

I included neurofeedback in my first book and found it very complex. For this book, I wanted to interview someone whose depth of knowledge would enable them to explain the treatment in simple terms anyone could understand. I phoned "The Brain Lady," Debra Burdick (covered later), asking who I should interview. She immediately recommended Mike Cohen,

Co-Founder of the Center for Brain in Jupiter, Florida, calling him the "national go-to-guy for neurofeedback."

"How is it," I asked Cohen, "that neurofeedback can treat so many different diagnoses?" The list of conditions it improves includes ADHD, addiction, anxiety/panic, autism, depression, cognitive dysfunction, epilepsy, head injuries, obsessive-compulsive disorder, PTSD/emotional trauma, and stroke.

"We don't treat the diagnoses," he explained. "We 'train' areas of the brain to be more efficient at their job, which often improves the symptoms of a variety of mental issues. For example, the temporal lobes regulate emotions. In many individuals with mental health issues, this would exhibit as a low tolerance for frustration. When frustration is a symptom, we train the temporal lobe area, and as functioning improves, the brain becomes more efficient at handling frustration." But before any training can begin, a comprehensive evaluation of each individual's brainwave patterns must be made.

At the Center for Brain, this evaluation is achieved by creating a brain map, also known as a qEEG (quantitative electroencephalogram). A qEEG is made by placing a snug cap on a patient's head. The hat contains 19 small electrodes measuring electrical activity from the brain, which is recorded by a computer and revealed on the monitor.

First developed at Brain Labs, part of the Medical School at New York University, brain mapping has been used for decades by advanced neurofeedback practitioners to help identify disorders of biological origin: schizophrenia, dementia, epilepsy, depression, brain atrophy, and attention deficit disorder. It has continued to progress in tandem with technology advances, but psychiatrists and mental health professionals usually do not use or recommend brain mapping. It is not part of their training and involves a huge new technical learning curve that most established practitioners would prefer to avoid.

Not all qEEG mapping services are alike, nor are all neurofeedback systems alike. There are simple plug-and-play neurofeedback systems that can be used after three hours of training, and there are extremely sophisticated systems requiring years to master but which are able to more precisely target a person's condition. This is why it is important to inquire about a practitioner's years of experience and expertise before making an appointment.

Following a qEEG, the brain map is evaluated by doing a statistical comparison of the results to a large database of how a normal brain should be functioning at this patient's age. After the assessment, treatment goals are established, and customized brain training begins, guided by the map results.

How a Brain Is Trained

Each training session involves placing electrodes on the head to measure brainwave activity, which is shown on the patient's monitor. There is no sensation of change in the brain, however. Patients simply watch the monitor and respond to "beep" audio tones that indicate they have received a "reward" for moving brainwaves toward a specific goal during that session.

To learn how to create this change, patients can select one of several fun, interactive feedback options: playing video games, manipulating sounds, watching movies, or moving real objects, such as slot cars. They are instructed to adopt a desired mental state: wakeful relaxation, intense focus, calm attention, meditative quiet, etc. As activity in the brain shifts in the desired direction, the interactive game progresses and the player scores, winning a reward. If brain activity does not change, or changes in an adverse direction, the game stops. Learning how to create a new brain wave pattern occurs gradually through trial and error, the instinctive way children learn. With repetition, brainwave patterns change, become habitual, brain functioning improves, and symptoms improve.

"The brain has an enormous capacity to repair itself," Mike Cohen told me. "Doing neurofeedback correctly requires targeting the specific problem area for each individual. Where it can become quite complex is when you're trying to identify and train the correct systems in the brain.

"One of the identification methods neurofeedback uses is by measuring brain activities and feeding this information back to the nervous system. Neurons fire between 1-200 times a second. If the brain is firing too much or too little, it is not working as efficiently as it should. Yet you do not feel neurons firing at all, so when neurofeedback brings a change in the firing pattern, you don't notice anything – you only become aware of changes by looking at the monitor.

"Neurofeedback is like a high-tech 'mirror' that tells your brain it's doing something," says Cohen. "The 'beep' of approval is mirroring back this success. Since the brain is a pattern-making machine, when you create an improved pattern and then the pattern stops, the brain starts firing additional neurons to fill in that gap, reproducing its more efficient activity. It's not magic. Anybody can do it! Think of neurofeedback as a high-tech gym for the brain. By 'working' the circuits, it gets stronger," he concludes.

How long does it take? Each person's challenge is unique, so the number of neurofeedback sessions required depends on the severity of their dysfunction. On-line sources indicate anxiety or insomnia may take 15-20 sessions; ADHD or learning disabilities 30-50.

By 2000, biofeedback therapy was covered by roughly half the major insurance companies for 40 conditions. Neurofeedback is still considered part of biofeedback so may be covered by some insurance plans. Ask your neurofeedback practitioner for an estimate of treatment costs, then telephone your health care provider before the appointment to determine if neurofeedback is covered.

The Brain Lady

Debra Burdick is a Licensed Clinical Social Worker and Board-Certified Neurofeedback Practitioner. She offered outpatient psychotherapy, mindfulness skills, and neurofeedback during her successful career. Now retired from private practice, she continues to author books and deliver accredited mindfulness seminars across the nation for PESI, LLC.

It seems life had an agenda for Burdick – she had a child, a husband, and a business partner with ADHD. She helped her family and thousands of clients, becoming an expert in the process. The list of ailments that can be helped by neurofeedback on her website is lengthy. She assisted people of all ages but was especially drawn to helping children, who call her "the brain lady."

Today her website, www.thebrainlady.com, is like a Fairy Godmother's basket of resources for ADHD kids. It offers several ADHD books and workbooks, numerous CDs with mindfulness meditations, and three-hour tele-training digital downloads. Burdick's comprehensive Home Study System for parents, *A Holistic Approach to Successful Children with Attention Deficit/Hyperactivity Disorder,* includes 11 CDs.

By visiting her website, kids, teens and adults can also receive the Brain Lady's free 3-part video and learn how to calm their mind and body, reduce stress, change the channel on worry and negative thoughts, relax into the present moment, and feel better immediately.

One of her recent books, *ADHD: Non-Medication Treatments & Skills for Children and Teens,* took the Gold award in Psychology at the 29th annual Benjamin Franklin awards. It was designed specifically for clinicians and parents seeking medication-free treatments and skills to empower ADHD children and teens to thrive. Selected by over 150 librarians, booksellers, and other experts as the top book in its category, it offers well-developed tools, techniques, activities, and handouts that can be used right away to treat ADHD without medications.

"Medication, which should be a last resort for kids with ADHD, has become the knee-jerk first and often the only offered treatment. This speaks to the crucial importance of Debra Burdick's latest book, *ADHD: Non-Medication Treatments and Skills for Children and Teens.* The book offers one hundred and sixty-two techniques, tips, activities and resources that can be used instead of medication to manage and moderate the worst ADHD symptoms. I highly recommend this book for parents, either dealing with a new ADHD diagnosis in a child or for those who wish to try another option other than medication."

--**Dr. Dale Archer**, Psychiatrist and NY Times bestselling author of *Better Than Normal* and *The ADHD Advantage*

Burdick's latest book, *Mindfulness for Teens with ADHD,* offers powerful skills to help kids successfully navigate all the areas of life: making good choices, completing tasks, increasing academic success, excelling at sports, driving safely, getting enough sleep, managing stress, and more. She maintains that by learning to pay attention in the moment, they'll be less distracted and better able to focus on what's going on right now—whether it's an algebra test, a job interview, or an important conversation with a friend.

Recent Research

I realize many ADHD patients find reading anything lengthy difficult. Start with Debra Burdick's website and books first. They provide practical, comprehensive, well-tested guidance.

For science fans, the link below leads to an article summarizing research on how neurofeedback works, with sections on its impact on ADHD, learning and developmental disabilities, cognitive and memory enhancement, uncontrolled epilepsy, traumatic brain injury and stroke, alcoholism and substance abuse, antisocial personality and criminal justice, posttraumatic stress disorder, autism and Asberger's Syndrome, anxiety and depression, insomnia, headaches and migraine, optimal performance training, and other clinical applications.

What is Neurofeedback: An Update, by D. Corydon Hammond, PhD, was published in 2011 to educate professionals and the general public. Dr. Hammond is Professor Emeritus at the University of Utah School of Medicine, Department of Physical Medicine and Rehabilitation. A trained Psychologist, he has advanced specialties in neurofeedback, quantitative EEG brain mapping, and clinical hypnosis. Here is a link to his complete review: http://dx.doi.org/10.1080/10874208.2011.623090

Resources:

Center for Brain: 550 Heritage Drive, Suite 140, Jupiter, FL, 33458, Tel 561 744-7616, https://www.centerforbrain.com/

Debra E. Burdick, author, speaker, mindfulness instructor, deb@thebrainlady.com.

PART III

TAPPING FOR RELIEF

CHAPTER 8

EMOTIONAL FREEDOM TECHNIQUE FOR PTSD, ANXIETY, AND EMOTIONAL TRAUMA

Energy psychology is a collection of mind-body approaches for improving human functioning. It focuses on the relationship between thoughts, emotions, sensations, and behaviors through bioenergy systems, such as meridians and the energy field encompassing our body. Emotional Freedom Technique (EFT) is the most well-known form of energy psychology due to its ease of use, speed, and effectiveness. It rapidly eases anxiety disorders, including phobias, as well as severe emotional trauma resulting from war, natural disasters, horrific accidents, rape, and incest.

The limbic system, one of the first parts of the brain to evolve, is the source of instinctive emotions and reactions. This primitive, rudimentary structure reacts more quickly than the rational brain to ensure survival, which is why people may become "irrational" in the midst of an accident or crisis. Any experience having high emotional impact is preserved in long-term memory, to help us respond more quickly to future threats. If trauma is experienced very early in life, or repeatedly over time, however, it may be stored in the subconscious. The emotional reactions persist but the source of them is not recalled. This is how old feelings and sensations continue to surface for years despite the reality that current circumstances do not pose a threat.

In the past, trauma has been primarily treated with talk therapy or psychiatric medications. Since these address symptoms rather than underlying causes, the trauma is never healed physiologically, and it self-perpetuates during prolonged talk therapy or when triggered by seemingly ordinary, related, or even unrelated events.

Research at Harvard Medical School has documented that the most effective treatment for trauma comes through energy psychology techniques, such as Emotional Freedom Technique (EFT/Tapping), Eye Movement Desensitization & Reprocessing (EMDR), and Therapy Acupoint Tapping (TAT). These all involve stimulating certain points on the body, which has been shown by MRI and PET scans to calm the amygdala in the brain and stop the fight or flight process from beginning. Research also reveals that the hippocampus and body's other fear sensors are similarly and often quickly affected. While memories are retained, they no longer carry an emotional intensity that triggers a trauma response. This enables full healing with respect to the originating event.

"Based on my clinical experience and reading of the research literature, EFT is the treatment of choice for rapid intervention in traumatic situations like Newtown, that trigger overwhelming emotions in individuals and groups. Its use can prevent the future development of full-blown PTSD by empowering people to develop control over their own nervous systems."

--Eric Leskowitz, MD, Department of Psychiatry, Harvard Medical School

Evolution of EFT

Stimulation of acupoints for psychological therapy began with Roger Callahan's development of Thought Field Therapy in the 1970s and continued evolving. Several variations now exist. The most popular form of EFT was created in the 1990s by Gary Craig, a Stanford engineer specializing in healing and self-improvement.

EFT is performed by physically tapping certain acupuncture junctions (acupoints) while voicing positive affirmations to relieve a specific problem—anxiety, a phobia, posttraumatic stress, and other sources of physical or emotional pain. EFT tapping releases emotional trauma and clears blockages along the bioenergy system. If the trauma was repressed, tapping releases it into consciousness where it can be processed in therapy. For a demonstration of EFT, go to http://www.youtube.com/watch?v=IWu3rSEddZI. Craig's EFT manual is available free at http://meridianvitality.com/gary-craigs-eft-manual/.

Even with EFT's long-standing history of success, three large pilot studies conducted between 2001 and 2005 met with strong professional criticism and incredulity because the speed of treatment and effectiveness rates of EFT far surpassed any previous method. Use persisted, however, due to EFT's astounding results and lower treatment costs, since it took only three to five sessions to resolve most long-standing emotional problems.

Finally, a December 2012 review of EFT by researcher David Feinstein, PhD, published in the American Psychological Association's journal, *Review of General Psychology*, found its protocols "consistently demonstrated strong effect sizes and other positive statistical results that far exceed chance after relatively few treatment sessions."

In the review, Feinstein describes the three early, large-scale pilot studies that were particularly provocative because of their speed and success rates for the conditions being studied. In one of these, a group of clinicians at Kaiser Permanente in Honolulu followed the progress of 714 patients being treated with EFT (Sakai et al., 2001). Patient reports of subjective distress showed statistically significant improvement for 28 presenting mental problems.

A second preliminary study emerged after Joaquín Andrade, a physician trained in acupuncture and EFT, brought acupoint tapping for psychiatric conditions to a group practice running 11 clinics in Argentina and Uruguay. In an ongoing in-house investigation, his team tracked the progress of 5,000 anxiety patients over a 5-1/2-year period. Improvement was found in 90% of the acupoint tapping group and 63% of the cognitive behavior therapy (CBT) group, with complete relief of symptoms at 76% for acupoint tapping and 51% for CBT.

Even more provocative was a third large-scale investigation by Carl Johnson—a retired Veterans Administration psychologist and a diplomat of the American Board of Professional Psychology. Johnson's initial report described his work with 105 people during his first five visits to Kosovo following the genocide, claiming strong improvement with 103 of them (Johnson et al., 2001). He went on to claim that 334 of 337 traumatized individuals—following treatment provided by him and his colleagues in Kosovo, Rwanda, the Congo, and South Africa—were able to bring to mind their most traumatic memories from the disaster and experience no physiological/affective arousal.

Feinstein concluded:

"A review of current evidence revealed that the use of acupoint stimulation in treating psychological disorders has been examined in a number of studies that met accepted scientific standards. These studies have consistently demonstrated strong effect sizes and other positive statistical results that far exceed chance after relatively few treatment sessions. Investigations in more than a dozen countries by independent research teams have all produced similar results. Speculation on the mechanisms involved suggests that tapping on acupoints, while a presenting emotional problem is mentally activated, rapidly produces desired changes in the neurochemistry involved in that problem. If favorable outcome research on energy psychology continues to accumulate—as recent developments would predict—and explanatory models for the observed effects continue to evolve, acupoint stimulation will offer clinicians a technique that can be used with confidence for quickly altering the neural pathways that underlie psychological problems."

As predicted, the latest 2016 meta-analysis completed for EFT treatment of PTSD continues to show outstanding results (Sebastian, B, Nelms, J, 2016, *Journal Explore Science and Healing*).

Thanks to this review, the APA approved the Association for Comprehensive Energy Psychology (ACEP) as a provider for continuing education credits in energy psychology and certification, welcoming it into mainstream medicine. For those who want more details and data, I recommend reading the full review by David Feinstein, which is available free at http://m.philmollon.co.uk/upload/Acupoint Stimulation Research Review%20(1).pdf.

Three Case Histories

Because most research is conducted using adult populations, I would like to share a few case histories that illustrate how EFT treatment takes place and can succeed with children. Suzanne Rossini, a Certified EFT Practitioner and Level 3 AAMET Certified Practitioner, sent the case-histories, which demonstrate how quickly kids respond. Rossini is a specialist in providing brain-based somatic relief techniques for trauma and other stress related issues in children, teens, and young adults. She is also a member of Tapping Star, an organization that encourages the use of Tapping for children in schools, institutions, parenting, and mentoring.

#1 Angelo, a 13–year–old boy with uncontrolled rage.
I first met Angelo in the spring of 8th grade. He had been having trouble with bullying and uncontrolled rage, which resulted in numerous detentions, a decline in his academic performance, and several school suspensions. Fortunately, an astute administrator recognized his symptoms as untreated trauma and referred Angelo to the Tapping Solution Foundation for treatment of PSTD.

Dr. Lori Leyden began addressing the effects that both the situation and a family history of domestic violence had on Angelo's ability to manage his rage. Using the gentle principals of EFT, Angelo was able to release the emotional charge of past events and respond with more control when triggered by a threatening situation. Although his behavior improved significantly, Angelo still had some remaining concerns about his ability to self-regulate anger. He also struggled with excessive weight and acid reflux, which he referred to as "the volcano of rage in my stomach." These were the symptoms we would explore together in the next 5 months.

My biggest challenge was allowing Angelo to manage the content while I managed the process. When adolescents share the content, they are often dismissive or unable to describe their feelings, especially if there are feelings of shame or embarrassment. This makes it difficult to determine points of emotional intensity and to measure progress. When asked about his emotional state (other than anger), Angelo would often answer with phrases like: "I don't really care" (translation: I care so much I can't even express it); "I was just annoyed" (translation: That's about as intense as I can get); or, "I don't know." When asked where he felt the emotion in his body, the answer was always, "in my stomach." The only time Angelo was able to describe and measure the intensity of his feelings was when he was angry. Then he often used superlatives like "off the Charts" and "the number is in the gazillions."

With each problem, I met Angelo where he was, used only his words, and measured his progress by observing subsequent actions. There were three "hot" areas: fear of managing rage, excessive weight, and acid reflux. Beginning with a physical symptom is a gentle approach, and I needed Angelo to feel safe releasing the rage that was stuck in his body. I decided to tackle acid reflux.

We began with his words: "Even though I have this acid reflux which is like a volcano of rage in my stomach and right now it's burning at a 5 … I'm a good kid and I'm doing the best I can." We do a round of tapping on the burning in the stomach and bring it down to a 2 level. Angelo has a cognitive shift and says: "This rage for my father in my stomach is off the charts." He does not appear agitated, but he clearly is ready to begin releasing some of his rage. I ask if he is able to rate the rage from 0-10 and he says 10. I tap down the intensity to a 2 using the set–up statement: "Even though this rage in my stomach for my Father is off the charts at a 10, I'm still a good kid and I'm doing the best I can."

I ask Angelo if he can remember a specific story with his Dad that still holds some intensity. He tells the story of a fight between his parents. Although there were many intense moments in the story, none of them were above a 2 for Angelo, except when he told about his Father not remembering the event the next morning. This enraged Angelo at a 10: "Even though my rage is off the charts because my Dad didn't even remember that fight … I'm still a good kid." We tap a round, but the intensity remains at a 10. I ask him what about his father's memory lapse most bothers him. He answers, "He didn't remember because he was drunk."

I decide to use this as the new set-up statement because it's more specific. I ask him if the intensity is still a 10 and he says no it's a 5 now, because his Dad had the excuse of being drunk. We tap this part of the story to a 2. I ask him how he knows the rage is at a 2 and he answers, "I don't know, it's confuziling. I don't know, and I can't think about it. I'm tired." It should be noted that the entire time Angelo was tapping he was yawning and stretching. You could almost see the energy moving in his body.

Angelo's rage episodes shifted from happening every other day to once every two months. He does not tap on his own, but he releases excess rage with a punching bag and by skate boarding. He reports the rage about his Father has diminished. His weekend visits are more enjoyable, since he and his Dad share some common interests. Telling the story has also greatly reduced Angelo's acid reflux. His mother reports he was able to stop the prescription medication and only occasionally needs over-the-counter relief. He started having symptoms when his first year of high school began and finds he still needs to visit the nurse occasionally.

Angelo's overwhelming anger and feelings of powerlessness at being bullied are absent, and instead of lashing out in rage he was able to report an incident to a teacher. In a period of several months he was transformed from a problem student to a leader.

#2 Christine, a 6-year-old girl with Autism Spectrum Disorder and severe expressive language problems

Christine has difficulty negotiating conflict with her classmates and, once angry, ruminates on the incident throughout the school day. She can be very oppositional about almost everything. Christine has superior art skills and loves to be read to. When her classmates do not include her in a game called "Zombie" they play at recess, this makes her extremely angry. She rates her anger at 11. When asked if she would like to tap about the incident she says, "No, my father says they shouldn't do this to me." (The teacher identifies this as a ruminating response.) When I ask Christine if she feels this anger anywhere in her body, she says no.

In spite of this resistance, Christine is able to demonstrate perfect tapping protocol and does so throughout the school day at random times. She is capable of repeating set-up statements verbatim that were previously used in group tapping lessons. She also exhibits excellent recall of all the tapping points. This incongruent behavior suggests that Christine is getting some relief from tapping but lacks the language skills necessary to articulate the problem. I suspect her perseverance serves to protect her in some ways but limits her ability to release anger. I am also concerned about her lack of kinetic awareness but will address this issue another time. The challenge here is to guide Christine gently to a place where she feels safe acknowledging and releasing her anger. I will use Christine's artistic skills to engage her throughout this experience.

When a child is resistant to tapping for any reason, you can do a little "sneaking-up" by using a tool known in EFT circles as "The Box." In this case, Christine does not want to tap about her anger, so The Box provides some protective distancing by creating a safe space to tuck away an event or feeling until the client is ready to acknowledge it. The Box can either be real or imaginary. In Christine's case, I know she is a wonderful artist, so I suggest she decorate a box to place her anger in. She loves this idea and decorates a crayon box with pink and blue hearts. (Cute choice for anger I think!) I help her write a set-up statement on an index card: "I am angry at an 11 about the 'Zombie Game' and my father says they shouldn't do this to me." We place the card in the box. The Box is also commonly used to gently close a session that may need more attention at a later date. I tell her we can look in the box tomorrow, and she is satisfied.

The next day I ask Christine if she would like to look in The Box. She happily gets her beautiful box and opens it. We read the index card and I ask her if she would like to tap about the "Zombie Game?" She says no. Christine is not ready to tap, so we place the index card back in the box.

I decide to offer another protective distancing strategy. There is an abundance of children's literature that targets the many emotional challenges children face. Using books helps them identify and acknowledge these challenges in a non- threatening way. I know Christine loves books, so I think this approach may work. I try to find stories that represent the presenting emotion. In this case, I select Molly Bang's book, *When Sofie Gets Angry, Really, Really Angry.* This is a wonderful story about a little girl who learns how to cope with her rage. My hope is that Christine will be inspired to manage her own anger. This strategy is successful, as the book provides many opportunities for discussion.

I ask Christine what number she thinks Sofia's rage is in the beginning of the story. She answers 11. I then ask her what number Sofia's rage is at the end of the story. She answers 5. I ask Christine if she would like to try tapping to help her with the anger she feels towards her friends. She is willing to a try, but requests to put the anger back in The Box whenever she wants to. We both agree. The tapping goes very well. Christine uses the set-up statement she wrote on the index cards and now rates her anger at a 5 (like Sofia), instead of 11. With a few rounds of tapping Christine gets to a 0. The anger is gone. I ask her how she knows it's gone. She answers, "I can play my own game." Christine then requests to sing the Yicky Yucky Song (a song we sing before the morning tapping circles class). The session ends with her singing and tapping on all the points. She is calm and happy.

Christine's cognitive shift, "I can play my own game," is quite remarkable given her problem with perseverance. It's important to monitor future experiences that present similar aspects of the original problem. I ask the teacher to observe her behavior. The following week her teacher reports that Christine's reaction is not as intense and in spite of being excluded she is able to continue her play either on her own or with other children. This tells me we are headed in the right direction. Although Christine continues to be a reluctant tapper, she is often seen tapping on the points throughout the school day without a direct request from the teacher. This response is consistent with her tendency to be oppositional. If you ask me to tap the answer will be no, but if you allow me to tap when I want, that's ok! Another example of meeting the child where they are.

My suggestions to Christine's teacher are: insist that she sit with the class for morning tapping circle but allow her the choice of tapping and continue to use books that gently open up discussions about feelings. Both these strategies have provided a safe bridge for Christine to release her anger and feel safe on the other side.

#3 Tom, a 5-year-old boy, lowers anger and frustration by tapping with a puppet

Teachers report that Tom thinks nothing he does is ever good enough. Even when his work is acceptable, he is unable to recognize it and refuses to continue working. His frequent tantrums often result in removing him from the classroom. When I ask him if this is a problem, he says "NO," but then nods his head "yes" and tells me he doesn't want to talk about it. I ask him to show me with his hands how angry he gets when teachers want him to finish his work, and his arms spread wide. Given his reluctance to speak about the problem, I use the class tapping dog, "Blaze," and ask him if it's ok for me to say the problem while he taps on Blaze. This works beautifully.

The set-up is, "Even though I never think my work is good enough and this makes me so mad when teachers want me to keep working... I'm still a good boy." While repeating the phrase, he completes three tapping sequences on the top of his head, top of eyes, side of eyes, under nose, on chin, a Tarzan thump, and monkey arms.

I ask Tom to create a book about himself that will include all the things he likes and does well. I say, "Let's both notice what happens when you feel your book isn't good enough, okay? Maybe I can help you feel more comfortable!"

As he works, he becomes frustrated with some of the pictures he draws, but he is able to work through these feelings tapping as we go. He completes a four-page book. I ask him to show me how angry he felt when he didn't like his picture. His hands come together. We tap about what a talented good boy he is!

Blaze sits in a special part of the room, and when Tom feels that anger, he is allowed to visit Blaze. The resource teacher reports that tapping on a regular basis has helped Tom complete his work more comfortably. The school psychologist is using calm and contain techniques (tap and breath/tap the inside of the ankle or wrist) with him, and reports his tantrums are less severe and shorter.

Resources:

Emotional Freedom Technique website: www.eftuniverse.com

EFT video demonstration http://www.youtube.com/watch?v=IWu3rSEddZI

Gary Craig's free EFT manual: http://meridianvitality.com/gary-craigs-eft-manual/

David Feinstein's full text 2012 article, published in *Review of General Psychology:* http://m.philmollon.co.uk/upload/Acupoint_Stimulation_Research_Review%20(1).pdf

EFT research: http://www.eftuniverse.com/research-studies/research

Suzanne Rossini, Certified EFT Practitioner, AAMET Level III, Tapping4peacect@gmail.com

Videos of children tapping: http://www.tappingstar.com

PART IV
Natural Nutrient Repairs

CHAPTER 9

AMINO ACIDS
FOR ALL TYPES OF ADDICTIONS

The brain registers all pleasure the same way, regardless of whether it results from a drug, alcohol, monetary reward, satisfying meal, or sexual encounter. The neurotransmitter dopamine creates the rush of pleasure we feel as it is released into a cluster of nerve cells beneath the midbrain's cerebral cortex. Dopamine also interacts with another neurotransmitter, glutamate, to aid learning and memory.

Reward-related learning sustains life by linking actions necessary for human survival, such as eating and sex, with pleasure and reward. However, the brain's reward system connects areas that stimulate motivation, memory, as well as planning and execution of tasks. This is the "pleasure circuit" that carries us from craving an intense pleasure to losing control over its use yet continuing to use it despite adverse consequences.

Dopamine is the neurotransmitter responsible for energy, emotions, movements, and an overall sense of well-being. It fuels cognition, memory, decision-making, and stress management. Motivation to exercise and complete tasks, as well as sensations of pain and pleasure, also depend on dopamine. Low levels are what drive addiction and contribute to other disorders.

Results of Low Dopamine:

Alcoholism
Attention deficit disorder
Drug abuse

Food bingeing
Internet addiction
Pathological gaming
Parkinson's disease
Sex addiction

Over time, the brain adapts to this dopamine flood, and it has less impact. Users need more of their addiction to get the same "high." As pleasure subsides, the memory of it and desire to repeat it persists, due to information stored in the brain that creates a conditioned response—intense cravings. This is why an addict may relapse after years of abstinence.

What if you could provide this rush of pleasure without the development of addiction? Dopamine is made from the amino acid Tyrosine. Amino acids are natural proteins contained in foods the body uses to produce all brain neurotransmitters. When supplements of concentrated forms of amino acids are given to addicts, their mood radically improves, sometime within a few minutes.

While amino acid treatments can be the beginning of life-long recovery and emotional stability, much of the scientific research documenting the chain reaction involved in addiction since the 1960s has been driven by one top addiction researcher, Dr. Kenneth Blum.

Early Amino Acid Therapy

By the 1980s, two pioneering holistic clinicians, Joan Mathews Larson, PhD, and Julia Ross, MA, MFT, learned of Blum's research and incorporated his use of concentrated blends of natural amino acids in their work with alcoholics and other addicts.

After the untimely death of her young husband, Larson became a single mother of three. Slowly she realized her sixteen-year-old son, Rob, was addicted to drugs and alcohol. She admitted him for a month into a Minneapolis hospital offering "state-of-the-art" treatment, which included reviewing the mistakes of his young life through daily counseling. After returning home, still filled with despair and hopelessness, Rob committed suicide. Larson realized, too late, that no amount of talk therapy could change the body chemistry creating his moods and cravings. She immersed herself in trying to understand the biochemical sources of depression, anxiety, irritability, and insomnia. She obtained a PhD in nutrition, opened an outpatient clinic in 1980 called Health Recovery Center (that is still in business), and authored *Depression-Free Naturally* in 1999.

Meanwhile in the San Francisco Bay area, Julia Ross, was working in residential psychiatric settings, leading therapy groups and workshops, and running treatment programs for adults and adolescents with addictions. As director of her first counseling program in 1980, she began to suspect poor nutrition was involved in the cases that did not respond to the intensive psychotherapy and spiritual support programs. Ross hired nutritionists to explore the possibility of a food-mood connection. They soon made a breakthrough.

Clients who were willing to eat plenty of protein and fresh vegetables three times a day, while avoiding caffeine, sweets, and refined starches (like white bread and pasta) felt much better emotionally and physically. Those who did not make the nutritional changes did not do nearly as well, despite lowering stress through exercise, long vacations, and moderate work hours. Yet, it took roughly ten weeks of following the healthy program for clients to withdraw from the bad-mood junk foods and fully experience the benefits.

Ross knew something was needed to speed up the process. Her search led to the work of Dr. Kenneth Blum. She added concentrated amino acid supplements into her nutritional therapy programs to increase the supply of "feel good" neurotransmitters. Her clients' recovery became quicker and more certain. Ross founded a successful holistic recovery clinic and authored two information-packed guides, *The Diet Cure* and *The Mood Cure,* before retiring.

Both women's clinics offered amino acid and natural nutrient protocols that successfully halted the powerful cravings of addiction. They agreed on the two primary causes of addiction: 1) inherited or stress-triggered nutrient deficits, and 2) inherited blood-sugar dysregulation, made worse by a junk food diet. Other biophysical causes they found associated with addictions included: low thyroid function, stress and adrenal burnout, unbalanced sex hormones, digestive dysfunction, and toxic overload. A study by Larson's Health Recovery Center in Minneapolis showed one-third to one-half of alcoholics treated also had pyroluria, a commonly inherited cause of mental illnesses discussed in Chapter 10.

Larson's book, *Seven Weeks to Sobriety,* describes a follow-up study of 100 Health Recovery Center alcoholic clients that showed 92% remained abstinent after six months. Three years after treatment, 95 people from the group were again interviewed, with 74% remaining clean and abstinent—numbers far surpassing the long-term recovery rate of 3-10 percent from 12-Step and other programs.

Taking specific amino acids became a successful part of nutrient treatments offering life-long recovery and emotional stability for addicts, but it has taken researchers many more decades to understand the complex science involved.

Researcher Kenneth Blum, PhD

Dr. Kenneth Blum, a top addiction researcher, led the way. In 1968, Blum and his mentor, Irving Geller, studied the role of neurotransmitters in stress and aberrant alcohol drinking. Their discovery that intense stress-related behavior in rodents was associated with reduced brain serotonin (a "feel good" neurotransmitter) became pivotal to the later development of an effective treatment.

At the University of Texas from 1972 through 1995, Blum proposed and researched many then-novel concepts, including the idea that alcohol craving is related to neurotransmitters and that the neurotransmitter dopamine can block withdrawal from alcohol. In 1989, Blum and colleague Ernest P. Noble, PhD, also made headlines with the discovery of the first gene associated with severe alcoholism (JAMA, April 1990).

Memory, learning, stress, and healing are all affected by classes of genes. Genes are activated by the environment inside a body—one's emotional, biochemical, mental, energetic, and spiritual landscape. The outer environment also impacts whether genes are "expressed" (turned on or off) and includes foods, toxins, social rituals, human and animal predators, even sexual cues. Dawson Church, PhD, in his revolutionary book, *Genie in Your Genes*, says researchers estimate that 90% of all genes are affected by signals from these environments. Dr. Blum went on to identify a few genes that could cause the brain to under-produce the "feed good" neurotransmitters and over-produce those that made people feel bad and be more vulnerable to addiction.

In 1995, Blum was the first to conceive of a group of conditions where low or inadequate levels of dopamine in the midbrain could cause addictive, obsessive, and compulsive behaviors, including attention deficit disorder, substance abuse, food bingeing, pathological gaming, internet addiction, and sex addiction. He coined the phrase "Reward Deficiency Syndrome" to refer to this concept. It has since been used in hundreds of peer-reviewed articles globally, and there is now a *Journal of Reward Deficiency Syndrome and Addiction Science.*

Work by Blum and colleagues in 1996 revealed a genetic aberration that leads to an alteration in the reward pathways of the brain. A variant form of the gene for the dopamine D_2 receptor, called the A_1 allele, was found. It was the same variant previously found to be associated with alcoholism. This time the researchers examined evidence suggesting that the A_1 allele was also associated with a spectrum of impulsive, compulsive and addictive behaviors. Blum concluded, "The concept of a reward deficiency syndrome unites these disorders and may explain how simple genetic anomalies give rise to aberrant behavior" (Blum, et al, *American Scientist*, 1996).

Synaptamine

Dr. Blum's career has been a decades-long quest to discover what drives addiction and how to successfully treat it. His work led to looking at all addictive, obsessive, and compulsive behaviors as *inherited, genetically-based illnesses,* not a slacker's choice or character flaw. Suddenly the big question became, "What is the best way to create dopamine balance in people involved in addiction treatment and recovery?" Blum had an answer, developed and tested in numerous clinical trials over the years and tweaked to perfection.

Synaptamine was launched in 2015 as an *affordable, easy-to-use, liquid supplement that can halt addictive cravings of any kind.* It regulates addictive cravings, supports optimum brain health, and promotes neurotransmitter balance, focus, and cognition, while increasing energy and reducing stress. It is the only all-natural single supplement available that *restores dopamine levels in the brain.* Non-addictive, it rarely causes side effects, which are mild and transient if they occur.

The supplement is an all-natural proprietary blend of precursor amino acids (the building blocks of neurotransmitters), vitamins, herbs, and other substances that support neurotransmission: Thiamine, Vitamin B6, Chromium polynicotinate; a fixed dose combination of amino acids and herbs called Synaptose, which contains DL-phenylalanine, L-tyrosine, Passion Flower extract; L-glutamine; 5-Hydroxytryptophan; Thiamine hydrochloride; Pyroxidal-5-phosphate; Pyridoxine HCI and a composite containing

Arabinogalactans, N-acetylglucosamine, Astragalus, Aloe Vera, Frankincense resin, White Pine bark extract, N-acetyl-cysteine, and Rhodiola.

The customary dose of Synaptamine is one-half ounce (1/2 capful) twice a day, the first before breakfast and the second before dinner (after a minimum two-hour protein fast). At this dose, one 30-ounce bottle costing $42.99, provides a month's supply. Classified as "medical food," a physician's prescription or recommendation is required for purchase. Online sources include:

> https://sanusbiotech.com
> http://lavitards.com/products/108/synaptamine
> http://holisticdrugrehab.com
> http://addictionsupplements.com/synapta/index.html

Opioids and Overdose Crises

The term opioid refers to a class of drugs that includes the illegal drug heroin, synthetic opioids such as fentanyl, as well as prescription pain medications oxycodone, hydrocodone, codeine, morphine, and many others. These drugs are all chemically related and interact with opioid receptors on nerve cells in the body and brain. They are well established as being addictive.

What has driven this relatively new epidemic? An increase in consumer demand for pain medications, partly from an aging population but also due to the pharmaceutical industry's enthusiastic promotion of these effective, extremely profitable, yet highly addictive pain killers. The rise in its use is outlined in the *American Society of Addiction Medicine's 2016 Opioid Addiction Facts & Figures report:*

- In 2010, sales of prescription pain relievers were four times the 1999 rate. (Pharmacies dispensed 69 tons of pure oxycodone and 42 tons of pure hydrocodone, enough to give 40 5-mg Percocets and 24 5-mg Vicodins to every person in the US.)
- In 2012, 259 *million* prescriptions were written for opioids, enough to give every American adult their own bottle of pills.
- By 2014, an estimated 21,000 adolescents used heroin, with 6,000 acquiring a heroin use disorder.

- Just a year later in 2015, 276,000 adolescents became current non-medical users of pain relievers; 122,000 of them had an addiction to prescription pain pills.
- Of the 20.5 million Americans 12 years or older who had a substance use disorder in 2015, two million used prescription pain relievers, while 591,000 took heroin.
- In 2015 the *leading cause of accidental death in the US* was 52,404 lethal drug overdoses.

In testimony before Congress on June 30, 2017, Dr. Wilson Compton, Deputy Director of the National Institute on Drug Abuse, reported the total "economic burden" of prescription opioid misuse alone in the US is estimated to cost $78.5 billion a year for health care, lost productivity, addiction treatment, and criminal justice involvement.

Synaptamine's proven success and economy should put it at the top of the list of treatments prescribed to combat this epidemic. Fifty dollars a month is far cheaper than most other treatment options and its use only requires a prescription, not a clandestine street buy. My concerns are whether medical practitioners will recommend something to patients that brings them so little income. And if not, how will patients/practitioners learn about Synaptamine, which has been available for two years yet seems relatively unknown.

Acupuncture Options

Since one treatment seldom suits every patient, acupunctrure is another option. Both the American College of Addictionology and Compulsive Disorders (ACACD) and the National Acupuncture Detoxification Association (NADA) have established acupuncture protocols that ease detoxification and withdrawal, reduce substance cravings, raise addiction program compliance, and relax patients by triggering feel-good endorphins.

The NADA protocol places traditional, fine stainless-steel needles under the skin for 45-60 minutes at five outer-ear points. The auricle, or outer-ear's microsystem, is also utilized by the ACACDs auriculotherapy, because it is the most direct neurological connection between the ear and brain. Instead of needles, however, ACACD's protocol uses a battery powered micro-current device, to stimulate *nerve endings* on the surface of the outer-ear. This more efficient process only requires a 10- to 20-minute treatment that normally costs $50-75 each. Although both protocols are effective, neither is considered a stand-alone solution. Once acupuncture treatment ceases, the patient's sense of well-being fades. Relapse is likely without dietary and lifestyle changes being made in conjunction with daily use of concentrated amino acid supplements to replenish neurotransmitter supplies and stabilize moods.

A comprehensive, natural biochemical approach for improving moods has been incorporated into the protocols of several addiction treatment centers in the US:

- **Alternative to Meds Center** in Sedona, Arizona, is a leading residential holistic mental health and addiction treatment center that combines Allopathic, Pain Management, Internal, and Environmental medicine with Naturopathic, Orthomolecular, and Chinese medicine. For 11 years it has helped thousands overcome withdrawal, instilling in clients a knowledge-and experienced-based, sustained recovery. www. alternativetomeds.com

- **InnerBalance Health Center** is a residential facility in Loveland, Colorado, that teaches clients to cope with symptoms, eliminate the source of cravings, and delivers lifelong tools necessary to stay sober. Extensive lab testing helps pinpoint and address biochemical causes: nutrient deficiencies; genetic factors; hormonal, adrenal, and amino acid imbalances; hypoglycemia; as well as toxic overload and the presence of heavy metals. www.innerbalancehealthcenter.com

- **Bridging the Gaps Inc.** in Winchester, Virginia, offers residential and out-patient treatment that begins with lab tests to assess liver and kidney function along with nutritional status. A psychological survey helps determine if clients are lacking certain brain chemicals. "Cocktails" of nutrients and amino acids are delivered intravenously, and clients are offered oral nutritional therapy and education, exercise, meditation, stress reduction techniques, and acupuncture. www. bridgingthegaps.com

- **Excel Treatment Center** in Denver, Colorado, is an outpatient service that specializes in providing intravenous nutritional therapy along with oral nutrients that help reverse genetic and drug related neurological damage. Intravenous therapy is administered in a painless drip over 3-4 hours for ten treatments, followed by weekly treatments for six months. Excel claims an 80% success rate over a 12-month period. www.exceltreatment.com

- **Community Addiction Recovery Association** (CARA) is a non-profit in Sacramento, California, treating chemical dependency with nutrition, supplements, acupuncture, acu-detox, herbal tea, and yoga. Staffed by licensed acupuncturists and certified clinical nutrition practitioners, a variety of mind-body integration techniques are also offered: https://www.sacramento365.com/organization/community-addiction-recovery-association/.

Correcting essential nutrient deficiencies and imbalances, improving one's diet, and taking specific concentrated amino acids is a well-established way to end addictive cravings for good, including the newest form, addiction to tech devices.

Technology Addictions

It's amazing how our lives have been transformed by technology in a relatively short time. Who would guess use of the internet, computer games, and cell phones could become addictive. What are some of the long-term effects screen addictions have on children, and what can be done (in addition to taking supplements) to control them?

An early study of internet addiction came from a 1998 Carnegie Mellon study. It found internet use over a two-year period was linked to increased depression, loneliness, and the loss of "real world" friends. In 2006, a Korean study of 1,573 high school students found a correlation between internet addiction, depression, and increased thoughts of suicide.

Dr. Nicholas Kardaras, PhD, LCSW-R, former Executive Director of the Dunes in East Hampton, NY, is one of the country's foremost addiction experts and author of *Glow Kids, How Screen Addiction is Hijacking Our Kids and How to Break the Trance.* Through his clinical work with over 1,000 teens in the last decade, Kardaras became aware that many were suffering from screen-addiction-triggered anxiety, depression, and psychosis-like symptoms. His desire to understand the impact of screen exposure on kids led to the discovery of research revealing that tech screens activate the brain's pleasure center as powerfully as sex. (Koepp et al, 1998)

The addiction is especially dangerous for younger children whose brains are still developing. One brain imaging study found the brains of video-gamers mirror damage done by drug addiction, contributing to abnormalities of myelin (white matter) in brain regions connected with executive attention, decision making, and emotional generation (Lei, Chinese Academy of Sciences, 2012). Brain imaging research on internet addicts showed compromised or "spotty" white matter, which leads to loss of communication within the brain. Impaired connections are believed to slow down or "short-circuit" signals and have been associated with ADHD, autism, addiction, and schizophrenia (Lin 2012, Yuan 2011, Hong 2013, and Weng 2013).

An Iowa State University study, co-authored by Dr. Dimitri Christakis, found that six- to 12-year-olds who spent more than two hours a day playing video games or watching TV had trouble paying attention in school and were 1.6 to 2.1 times more likely to have attention problems (*Pediatrics*, 2010). According to Dr. Christakis, an earlier study showed the more TV a child watches between the ages of one and three, the greater the risk of developing an attention problem by age seven (*Pediatrics*, 2004). She believes the pacing of programs, whether on video games or television, is over stimulating and contributes to the attention problems.

A 2010 Kaiser Foundation study found that elementary-aged kids use a daily average of eight hours of entertainment technology, 75% of them have televisions in their bedrooms, and 50% of North American homes have the TV on all day. Kids now rely on technology for the majority of their play, which limits expansion of creativity and imagination as well as important sensory and motor development. Chaotic sensory stimulation combined with a sedentary lifestyle also inhibits children from reaching important developmental milestones and obtaining basic foundational literacy.

The impact of technology on a developing child indicates that while their sense of body position in space, tactile sensations, and attachment systems are all under-stimulated, their visual and auditory senses are definitely on "overload." Kids who are exposed to violence through TV and video games are perpetually in fight-or-fight stress mode while watching or playing the game. Their body does not know that what they are watching is not real but simulated activity, so it continuously triggers adrenaline to prepare them for action. Thus, the body is always "on alert," waiting for the oncoming assault from video game characters. Such sensory imbalance disrupts neurological development as the brain's anatomy, chemistry, and pathways become impaired by stress.

Dr. Craig Anderson, Distinguished Professor of Psychology at Iowa State University, conducted the largest, most comprehensive meta-study review ever done of research on video games and aggression. He analyzed 130 studies with over 130,000 participants worldwide. The study found that violent games are not just related to but were also a causal risk factor for increased aggressive thoughts and behavior. Anderson stated, this "proves conclusively that exposure to violent video games makes more aggressive, less caring kids – regardless of their age, sex or culture" (*APA Journal Psychological Bulletin*, 2010).

Glowing screens are only part of the problem according to Chris Rowan, BScBi, BScOT, AOTA Approved Provider, and noted pediatric occupational therapist who has witnessed dramatic changes in how children are developing today. "They used to play outside all day, riding bikes, playing sports, and creating games. They moved a lot, with their sensory world nature-based and simple…. They ate meals together and talked about their day, developing strong connections," she says. The rapid rise in technology has fractured peer and family connections, eroding core values that once held them together.

"The virtual world is devoid of touch, movement, human connection, and nature – four critical elements for child development and learning," continues Rowan. "One in three children now enter school developmentally delayed, one in four are obese, one in six have a diagnosed mental illness, and one in ten are addicted to video games and/or pornography."

Rowan has developed a concept called Balanced Technology Management, where parents strive to create balance between tech-use and tech-free activities children need for growth and success. Her website (see resources) offers parents four tools to help find this crucial balance.

Tech Tools for Withdrawal
Technology Screen, a one-page grid for completion to help determine a child's baseline technology use rates.

Ten Steps to Unplug Children

1. become informed
2. disconnect yourself
3. reconnect with your kids during times set aside for "no technology"
4. explore alternatives to technology as a family
5. enhance performance skills *prior* to unplugging
6. meet developmental milestones by engaging in movement, touch, and connection
7. address fear of the dangers when kids play out-of-doors
8. create individual roles and foster independence within the family context
9. set a schedule that balances technology use and other activities
10. link tech corporations with communities to build sustainable futures for children

Technology Schedule, a weekly grid to schedule time for favorite TV programs, video games or internet activities, ensuring that it stays within the family-allotted daily/weekly tech use limitations.

Tech Diet – Is your family "tech fat?" A four-step plan to wean a family off technology:

- Rate – technology use
- Reset – unplug all technology
- Reorder – schedule activity replacement
- Rules – structure change

Addiction Research

For readers who enjoy science, dozens of clinical trial results are available through this link to an Open Access 2012 study. It summarizes what is known about dopamine deficiency and how Dr. Blum's all-natural supplement helps increase dopamine levels and end addiction: **https://www.ncbi.nlm.nih.gov/pmc/articles/PMC3733258/.**

For additional clinical trial data by population type (cocaine, alcohol, etc.), go to **http://addictionsupplements.com/synapta/index.html.**

Resources:

Health Recovery Center in Minneapolis, Joan Mathews Larson, PhD, Founder; author of *Seven Weeks to Sobriety*, **www.healthrecovery.com**

The Mood Cure **website of Julia Ross https://www.moodcure.com/find_practitioner.html,** listing mood specialists, addiction specialists, integrative psychiatrists in the US and abroad

Synaptamine addiction supplement, https://sanusbiotech.com/3731 W 10400 South, Suite 102-416, South Jordan, UT 84009, Tel 877 411-4397, **support@sanusbiotech.com**

ACACD Auriculotherapy, American College of Addictionology and Compulsive Disorders, **www.acacd.com**

Auriculotherapy Intro video, Part 1 (10 minute) **http://www.youtube.com/watch?v=Wd6y3dfyOyA**

Amino acids and auriculotherapy for addiction, video by Dr. Stokes (10 minute) **http://www.youtube.com/watch?v=B8Qr339uFIY**

Technology addiction research, http://drkardaras.com/

Alternative to Meds Center in Sedona, Arizona, Tel 1 800 301-3753, **www.alternativetomeds.com**

InnerBalance Health Center in Loveland, Colorado, Tel 1 800 900-2252, **https://innerbalancehealthcenter.com**

Bridging the Gaps Inc. in Winchester, Virginia, **www.bridgingthegaps.com**

Excel Treatment Center in Denver, Colorado, **www.exceltreatment.com**

Community Addiction Recovery Association in Sacramento, California, **www.carasac.org**

Chris Rowan, BScBi, BScOT, CEO Zone'in Programs, Inc. and Sunshine Coast Occupational Therapy, Inc., 6840 Seaview Rd., Sechelt, BC CANADA VON3A4; Tel 604-885-0986; websites: wwwzonein.ca, www.suncoastot.com, www.virtualchild.ca

CHAPTER 10

NUTRIENT POWER
FOR SCHIZOPHRENIA AND ALL MENTAL DIAGNOSES

By this point you have become familiar with several drug-free mental health treatments that may be new to you. All offer a realistic hope for recovery from diagnoses that are often considered "incurable" by conventional medicine. This chapter will primarily focus on using an "Orthomolecular" all-natural nutrient therapy for treating schizophrenia, although the method is also used to treat other mental dysfunctions. Simply taking specific nutrients prescribed for me based on lab testing that reveals each person's unique biochemistry, has kept my bipolar mood swings in check for 16 years. Schizophrenia, Autism, and Alzheimers are equally challenging yet often helped by the Orthomolecular protocol.

Parts of this chapter may be difficult to understand despite my attempts to make it simple. After a quick read, most details will quickly fade. What I hope you recall is that this approach has a 50-year history of bringing sustained improvements that often enable *schizophrenic patients to recover and enjoy "normal" lives* (described in a few case histories below). That alone makes it memorable and certainly worth trying.

Due to the complex science involved, it is important to find doctors trained in the use of natural substances for healing. Using the following titles or key words in an internet search will help locate holistic practitioners in your community: Naturopathic Doctors (ND) are trained to use natural nutrients, herbs, homeopathy, and other drug-free treatments; Functional doctors (MDs and NDs) often obtain training and certification in use of acupuncture, alternative, complementary, or Orthomolecular medical protocols.

Schizophrenia Idiosyncrasies

First described by the ancient Egyptians, schizophrenia now occurs in 0.3 percent of people around the world and includes 3.5 million US residents. A chronic, severe mental disorder, schizophrenia affects how a person thinks, feels, and behaves. Its symptoms can be very disabling: hallucinations, delusions, paranoia, and dramatic personality changes. Symptoms also include reduced facial expressions, feelings of pleasure, or ability to focus or speak, as well as trouble understanding information and using it to make decisions.

Symptoms usually become apparent between the ages of 15 and 25 in men and the ages of 16 and 35 in women. This diagnosis is especially frightening, because symptoms rapidly worsen, often causing patients to drop out of school, preventing them from keeping a job or living independently for the rest of their lives.

The first genetic family study of schizophrenia was conducted by Ernst Rüdin before World War I and published in 1916. Convincing twin studies over several decades revealed it to be a highly inheritable trait. If both parents are schizophrenic, the risk factor of having the disorder is around 37 percent. The highest risk, 57 percent, is found in individuals whose identical twin has schizophrenia, according to The Genetics of Mental Disorders (1971, Oxford University Press, London). However, researchers then and now acknowledge that dietary and environmental factors are also involved with the action of genes, although they do not yet fully understand how.

Psychosis is a severe mental state in schizophrenia where thoughts and emotions are so impaired that patients lose contact with external reality. Powerful drugs have been used successfully since the 1950s for calming and reducing psychosis. However, drug side effects – sedation, impaired cognition, socialization deficits, altered personality, movement disorders, diabetes, weight gain, and strokes – add to the physical and emotional challenges each patient faces.

The Orthomolecular approach to treating mental diagnoses was pioneered in the 1960s by two Canadian psychiatrists, Abram Hoffer, MD, and Humphrey Osmond, MD. To help family members and other physicians understand how these challenging symptoms can be halted or reduced, Hoffer later founded the International Society for Orthomolecular Medicine. Its annual conferences (www.orthomed.org) continue to educate consumers and practitioners. One US practitioner who adopted the Orthomolecular approach 30 years ago was Dr. William Walsh.

William J. Walsh, PhD

Walsh is an internationally recognized expert in the field of nutritional medicine and the man responsible for ending my bipolar symptoms. In 2011, he sold the clinic where I was treated to focus on his non-profit laboratory, Walsh Research Institute. In addition to conducting research, it regularly offers international physician training programs covering advanced biochemical/nutrient therapies in Australia, Norway, and other countries.

The author of over 200 scientific articles and reports, Walsh obtained degrees from Notre Dame and the University of Michigan along with a PhD in chemical engineering from Iowa State University. While working at Argonne National Laboratory in the 1970s, he organized a prison volunteer program that led to studies of prisoners and ex-offenders that helped determine the causes of violent behavior. Over time, he assembled a large database of the unique kinds of biochemistry that drives violence.

This research, combined with Walsh's later collaboration with Carl C. Pfeiffer, M.D., Ph.D., another Orthomolecular pioneer, led to the founding of an outpatient clinic outside Chicago in 1989. For two decades it enjoyed success improving the biochemistry of more than 25,000 people suffering from autism, schizophrenia, and Alzheimer's, as well as behavioral, attention deficit, mood, and anxiety disorders.

After the clinic closed, Walsh finally found time to write a book in 2012 describing this method of treatment. *Nutrient Power, Heal Your Biochemistry and Heal Your Brain* includes a 20-page chapter on schizophrenia, along with chapters on other major mental disorders. In a review, Marguerite Kelly, syndicated columnist for *The Washington Post*, said "This is the book that will revolutionize psychiatry.... If I could add a sixth star to this review, I would."

Walsh Schizophrenia Theories

Schizophrenia has frustrated researchers and practitioners for decades. Thanks to their persistence, it is now understood that the confusion comes from many different types of schizophrenia residing under this "umbrella diagnosis."

"Genotypes" are sets of genes in our DNA responsible for a particular trait, while "phenotypes" refers to the physical expression or characteristics of that trait. In the 1980s, Dr. Pfeiffer identified three different phenotypes of schizophrenia, each named after its cause: overmethylation, undermethylation, and pyrrole disorder. Based on blood and urine testing of 3,600 schizophrenic patients, Dr. Walsh expanded the list to include "gluten intolerance" and "other." He also identified five less-common causes in his book: porphyria, homocysteinuria, thyroid deficiency, cerebral allergy, and drug-induced schizophrenia. According to Walsh, among the five different schizophrenia phenotypes, 20% have pyrrole disorder, 42% overmethylate, 28% undermethylate, 4% are gluten intolerant, and 6% have other causes.

After years of studying the biochemistry of schizophrenic patients, Dr. Walsh has five theories about its root causes that fall into three categories.

Oxidative Stress

- **Walsh Theory #1** Predisposition to schizophrenia involves fetal programming errors that cause lifelong vulnerability to oxidative stresses.
- **Walsh Theory #2** The mental breakdown event is triggered by overwhelming oxidative stress that alters DNA and histone marks that regulate gene expression.

High oxidative stress in the brain is a distinctive feature of schizophrenia, with brain cell loss one indicator. Many researchers believe high oxidative stress may be *the primary cause* of schizophrenia and result from inherited, weak antioxidant protection by the body. It may be increased by the presence of heavy metals, viruses, bacteria, inflammation, injury, emotional stress, nuclear radiation, or high iron levels.

Epigenetic Changes

- **Walsh Theory #3** Epigenetic changes are responsible for continuing psychotic tendencies after the breakdown event, which is why the condition does not go away.
- **Walsh Theory #4** Failure to follow classical laws of genetic inheritance results from the epigenetic nature of schizophrenia.

Epigenetics is the study of potentially inherited changes in gene expression *that do not involve changes to the genetic code in our DNA.* When genes are said to be "expressed," it means they are either turned on or turned off, activated or silenced. "Phenotypes have now been broken into further subtypes, all due to epigenetics determined before you were born," says Walsh.

Methyl and folate levels are known to have a powerful epigenetic role in determining which genes are turned on or turned off, and abnormal blood levels of methyl and folate are present in about 70% of all schizophrenic patients. This explains how schizophrenia may run in families but not follow the classical laws of genetics. In many studies of identical twins, only one develops schizophrenia. Decades of research have not yet identified any genes responsible for schizophrenia. An important clue emerged, however, from the study of identical twins that found *epigenetic DNA methylation abnormalities* in the schizophrenic patients but not in their twin brothers.

Three Epigenetic Phenotypes

- **Walsh Theory #5 Three major phenotypes of schizophrenia develop in individuals who exhibit overmethylation, undermethylation, or overwhelming oxidative stress (also called pyrrole disorder).**

Undermethylation. Methylation is a critical biochemical process (one of the detoxification pathways) that happens over a billion times a second in your body. Roughly 28% of schizophrenia patients undermethylate and have severely depressed methyl/folate ratios. "If a person is undermethylated and you give them folate," says Walsh, "their status will improve dramatically. However, if you have a bipolar, schizophrenic, or violent person, they are totally intolerant of folate. Epigenetics solves this mystery." Folates have powerful genetic effects. They are a serotonin promoter and help inhibit reuptake of serotonin in the brain.

Although the dominant symptom of undermethylated schizophrenia is usually delusions, mild hallucinations are sometimes present. In general, these individuals are high achievers, and most of those experiencing mental symptoms respond to methylation therapies.

87

Case History - Nutrient Treatment for Undermethylation

David was a brilliant 22-year-old PhD candidate at Berkeley who developed disturbing symptoms after breaking up with his girlfriend. He stopped attending classes, told friends that Russian agents were trying to kill him, and would sit for hours with a blank expression. Diagnosed with schizoaffective disorder, he was hospitalized for ten days and medicated with Zyprexa, Depakote, and Zoloft. Despite significant improvement, David was unable to resume his studies or hold a job. He reported a 50-pound weight gain and isolated himself from his friends. A biochemical evaluation revealed symptoms of undermethylation. His blood histamine level was extremely elevated at 170 ng/ml, and he was treated with SAMe, methionine, calcium, magnesium, zinc, serine, and vitamins A, B-6, C, D, and E. His family reported no change for six weeks, followed by slow improvement. After a year of nutrient therapy, David reported a nearly complete recovery, and his psychiatrist weaned him from Depakote and Zoloft, reducing the dosage of Zyprexa. He has held a job as a computer specialist for the past five years.

Overmethylation. According to Walsh, overmethylation is the dominant chemical imbalance for about 42% of people diagnosed with schizophrenia. This phenotype features excess activity at dopamine and norepinephrine neurotransmitter receptors, possibly caused by epigenetic inhibition of dopamine and norepinephrine transporters, along with elevated copper levels. Commonly diagnosed as paranoid schizophrenia, the primary symptoms include auditory hallucinations, severe anxiety, paranoia, and agitation with high physical activity.

Case History - Nutrient Treatment for Overmethylation

Judy W, age 26, was a working nurse when she developed a sleep disorder, followed by high anxiety, a collapse in work performance, and auditory hallucinations. She reported a persistent condemning male voice telling her she was worthless and should kill herself. Judy received a leave of absence, saw a psychiatrist, and did weekly counseling as well as group therapy with little improvement. After being hospitalized for a week, she was prescribed Zyprexa, Tegretol, and Zoloft, which reduced hallucinations and allowed her to sleep. Her maternal grandmother had a history of severe anxiety and depression. As a child, Judy underachieved in school but had many friends. Her metabolic testing revealed a very depressed blood histamine level of 10 ng/ml, and she was diagnosed with over-methylation. Lab tests also showed elevated copper and depressed zinc levels. Nutrients prescribed were folic acid, zinc, niacin, and vitamins B-6, B-12, C, and E, all taken with her medications. The goal was to reduce her norepinephrine and dopamine levels while increasing GABA. Judy experienced a worsening of anxiety the first three weeks, followed by clear improvement during month two. Within six months, her symptoms were nearly gone, and she returned to work after a year's absence. Weaned off from Tegretol and Zoloft, she continues on a low dose of Zyprexa. (Excerpted from *Nutrient Power* with the author's permission.)

Pyrrole Disorder with high oxidative stress impairs brain functions and leaves people unable to cope with stress. The problem begins with overproduction of the HPL (hydroxyhemoppyrrolin-2-one) molecule during synthesis of red blood hemoglobin. Normally when the body overproduces something, it dumps the excess. Unfortunately, both zinc and vitamin B-6 are attracted to the HPL molecule, bond onto it, and are eliminated from the body too, causing a life-long deficiency of two nutrients essential to general health and brain function.

Zinc is required for a robust immune system, the production of 60 enzymes and neurotransmitters, use of amino acid proteins, and to maintain gut integrity. Vitamin B-6 is part of more than 2,000 different enzymes involved in digestion and metabolism, plus it is required for production of the "feel good" neurotransmitters serotonin, dopamine, and GABA. Vitamin B-6 deficiency can also impair short-term memory, contributing to academic underachievement.

Diagnoses of Pyroluria occur in:

11% of the general population
71% of patients with Down's syndrome
59-80% of patients with acute schizophrenia

40-50% of patients with chronic schizophrenia
47-50% of patients with bipolar mania/depression
12-46% of patients with major depression
46-48% of patients with autism
40-47% of patients with ADHD/ADD and learning disabilities
20-84% of patients with alcoholism
71% of patients with acute onset as adult criminals
33% of patients who are young violent offenders
(Source, Walsh Research Institute)

Case History - Nutrient Treatment for Pyrrole Disorder

Mary became head of a successful family business at age 29. Three years later, she suffered a severe mental breakdown when her mother died in an auto accident. After many unsuccessful medication trials, she became suicidal. Lab testing revealed several symptoms of pyrrole disorder, including morning nausea, aversion to sunlight, absence of dream recall, history of severe sunburn, preference for spicy foods, and abnormal menstrual cycles. She also exhibited classic pyroluric fat distribution, with concentrations at her midsection and upper thighs. Lab testing showed a urine pyrrole level exceeding 150 μg/ml, more than 10 times the normal level. Her nutrient therapy involved very high doses of zinc and vitamin B-6 together with augmenting nutrients. The family reported great improvement within 30 days, and at her three-month follow up evaluation she appeared completely recovered despite taking no psychiatric medications. She resumed her role as leader of the family business but suffered two serious relapses when she temporarily stopped the nutrient program. She and the business have done well since. (Excerpted from *Nutrient Power* with author's permission.)

Mensah Medical

After Dr. Walsh focused on research and teaching other doctors, two of his staff, Albert Mensah, MD, and Judith Bowman, MD, opened their own clinic, Mensah Medical, to serve those currently using the nutrient protocol along with new patients.

Dr. Mensah received his undergraduate degree from Northwestern University and his medical degree from Finch University of Health Sciences-Chicago Medical School. As a physician in a specialized field, he has treated over 3,000 patients with advanced targeted nutrient therapy since 2005. He also serves on the Board at Walsh Research Institute and as a clinical instructor for Walsh Research Institute's international doctor training programs.

I asked Dr. Mensah how Orthomolecular nutrient treatments had changed in the past decade. "Tremendous change," he said. "Now we understand the biotypes of schizophrenia. In early days, there wasn't any biochemical testing. Lab tests of blood and urine now determine which categories patients belong in and their treatment." Which lab tests are typically ordered for schizophrenia patients? "Histamine and pyrrole levels, hair analysis to identify gut issues, malabsorption of nutrients, and cellular stability. Without cellular stability, you can't have normal brain function," he says.

Do they use challenge urine testing to detect the presence of metals, such as lead? "When metals are sequestered in organs, they produce specific organ damage. You would not be seeing global effects unless those metals are out in circulation," he replied. "You cannot talk about metals as a singular group. Each has its own unique capacity, trouble, and protocol. Mercury has a half-life of 45 days. After a few months, whatever mercury you have consumed, it may be there, but it's not active. What happens with metals is they create inflammation when they come into your system. That is not fixed by removing the metals but by use of antioxidants. However, metals are not big causes of schizophrenia."

Asked about other discoveries, Dr. Mensah replied, "Many people don't know about the protein metallothionein (MT). A study showed higher levels of zinc than normal in the brains of Alzheimer's individuals. Researchers made the assumption it was causing Alzheimer's. They didn't know that when MT is in the brain, it goes there to regulate metals, and it uses zinc as fuel. The more zinc you see in Alzheimer's, the harder MT is working to help the patient."

When asked about research indicating that psychotic symptoms might be caused by a faulty "switch" within the brain, Mensah replied, "Lots of fabulous work going on. There are many switches in the brain. One is the N-methyl-D-aspartate (NMDA) receptor. The other switch involves oxidative stress overload. Trauma, rape, brutalization, or staying up late for several nights in a row all produce oxidative stress, tipping a once normal person into schizophrenia. The wonderful thing about switches is when something is turned on, it gives us a clue on how to turn it off. Natural elements in amino acids can be used to trip that NMDA switch. Dr. Hoffer would be thrilled."

Judith Bowman, MD, received a BA from Illinois Wesleyan University and a medical degree from Finch University of Health Sciences-Chicago Medical School. Certified and licensed by the American Registry of Radiologic Technology and board certified in Nuclear Medicine Technology after training at Northwestern University's School of Nuclear Medicine, she utilized her diagnostic imaging skills to participate in research and development of radio pharmaceuticals. Dr. Bowman was a staff physician for Lake County Health Department in Illinois and provided medical services for patients with learning disabilities at The Dore Achievement Center in Illinois before joining Dr. Walsh's team in 2005.

I asked Dr. Bowman, a skilled diagnostician, how her background in Nuclear Medicine helped. "When patients bring brain scans from other clinics, I can look at them and determine what's going on. I also participated in early studies of brain mapping using radio isotopes, which helps me understand what's happening in the brain during certain activities."

What should patients expect in an initial meeting for balancing biochemistry at Mensah? Patients are welcomed by a receptionist who gives them an overview of how the doctors work. A nurse records their family mental history and personal information covering their entire health history, followed by a review of symptoms and diagnosis, which requires 30-45 minutes. Doctors greet the patients and interview them for 45-60 minutes, to obtain more details and order lab testing. "We encourage them to actively participate in their treatment, to give us a monthly report on what they're experiencing via email or a visit, and to ask questions," says Bowman. "Our patients return (for evaluation) every six months the first year, or sooner if something difficult arises."

When asked what behaviors might cause her to order a particular lab test, Bowman replies, "Eating disorders. Any of the three eating disorders stems from undermethylation. Pyrrole disorder often comes with this too. These patients are mostly female perfectionists looking for a certain image, except that image is a delusion." The doctors check a patient's biochemistry and address the imbalances. Within 6-9 months, their behavior changes and they leave the delusional state and function better. "Counseling, psychotherapy, cognitive behavior therapy, or neurofeedback should be in the mix too," she says. "It's hard to unlearn those old habits."

Women's health is Bowman's other passion, especially psychotic behavior caused by estrogen dominance and high copper levels. "People don't connect the dots between anxiety, depression, or even psychosis and high levels of copper or estrogen," she says. Both can accumulate over time. "With the first baby, copper will be really high. It comes in like a flood to support the growth of blood vessels for the child. We hope it will go back to normal, but if she cannot excrete copper properly, it will go higher." By the third child, it will be sky high and the mother will develop post-partum psychosis and do "strange things, like shooting someone or walking off a building, all due to excess copper."

Visualize the brain as a typical copper-top battery. The components in a battery are potent metals in specific proportions. "When you put it into a toy, it works fabulously, but when it loses potency over time and starts to leak, the balance is lost," Bowman says. "This leads to dysfunction, cognitive disarray, bipolar and other symptoms caused by oxidative stress. Metallothionein (MT) is a protein made in the gut that gives the right proportions of minerals and metals." This is one of many ways nutrient power restores mental health.

New Areas of Research

Testing schizophrenia biotypes for epigenetic profiles. A key element missing in most research is recognition that schizophrenia is an "umbrella" term used to describe a variety of disorders. Walsh Research Institute and Queensland University of Technology (QUT) in Australia have formed a collaborative effort to analyze the DNA methylation characteristics of each schizophrenia biotype – an innovative first. Success could lead to identification of persons at risk for developing schizophrenia, creating prevention strategies, and designing improved biotype treatments. Cancer researchers have developed effective ways of identifying cancer-prevention genes that have been "turned off" by environmental insults and are developing therapies to restore proper gene function. The Queensland/Walsh collaboration's objective is to determine if a similar approach holds promise for schizophrenia.

Is abnormal brain development caused by excessive "pruning?" Early prenatal development of the prefrontal cortex is a period of high cellular proliferation. Animal models show that curtailing such growth produces schizophrenia-like pathology and mimics behavioral and cognitive symptoms of the disease. Social situations that elevate stress in adolescence also increase dopamine stimulation, which may lead to exaggerated synaptic pruning. In animal primates, dopamine hyper-stimulation decreases prefrontal pyramidal cell spine density and is associated with profound cognitive dysfunction. Thus, both gestation and adolescence are seen as two periods of human vulnerability for developing schizophrenia (Selemon LD, Transl Psychiatry, 2015).

Mental disorders may be brain circuit disorders. In 2005, the suggestion that mental disorders could arise from disruptions in the circuitry map of a developing brain was put forth by researchers studying genes, the proteins they produce, and their functions. As key factors that increase the risk of mental disorders were identified, a list was made of previously unknown proteins that had one thing in common: they are important for healthy brain development. In 2010, Tom Insel, MD, then Director of the National Institute of Mental Health wrote, "Unlike neurological disorders which often involve areas of tissue damage or cell loss, mental disorders have begun to appear more like circuit disorders, with abnormal conduction between brain areas rather than loss of cells." Neuroimaging technology has revealed that specific brain pathways, mostly in the prefrontal cortex, are involved.

A faulty "switch" in the brain is discovered. University of Nottingham research published in 2013 showed that psychotic symptoms experienced by people with schizophrenia might be caused by a faulty "switch" in the brain. The four-year study centered on the insula region, a segregated "island" deep in the brain responsible for seamless switching between the inner and outer world.

Research Fellow Dr. Lena Palaniyappan said, "We constantly switch between our inner, private world and the outer, objective world. This switching process appears to be disrupted in patients with schizophrenia. This could explain why internal thoughts sometime appear as external objective reality, experienced as voices or hallucinations." Functional MRI (fMRI) imaging was used to compare the brains of 35 healthy volunteers with those of 38 schizophrenic patients. While the majority of healthy patients were able to make the switch between regions, schizophrenia patients were less likely to shift to using their frontal cortex. Using fMRI to detect the lack of positive influence from the insula to the frontal cortex also appears to be a valuable diagnostic tool (Liddle P, Palaniyappan L, *Neuron*, August 2013).

Additional research on mental diagnoses, brain synapses, and circuits can be found at www.pubmed.gov.

In closing, I would like to share the sentiments of researcher Patrick F. Sullivan, MD, FRANZCP, a medical geneticist at the University of North Carolina School of Medicine:

"In psychiatry, we are at the end of the beginning, not the beginning of the end, and we will need more scientific cooperation, a more-clever research strategy, and higher statistical rigor in order to get a complete picture of schizophrenia neurobiology."

And may we make *restoring our children's mental health* the goal of all treatments.

Resources:

International Society for Orthomolecular Medicine, www.orthomed.org

Annual International Orthomolecular Medicine Conference: www.cimadoctors.ca/event/orthomolecular-medicine-today

Walsh Research Institute, 1155 S. Washington St, Naperville, IL 60540, Tel 630 364-2600, www.walshinstitute.org

Mensah Medical, 4355 Weaver Pkwy #110, Warrenville, IL 60555, Tel 630 256-8308, www.mensamedical.com

APPENDIX A

THE FOUNDATIONS OF HEALTH

Healthy Foods

The fuel our bodies need to generate energy, make repairs, and run internal systems comes from the intake of foods, fluids, and oxygen. Since staying healthy usually leads to lower medical costs and a more comfortable, enjoyable life, this made finding the best quality sources a top priority for me.

Many years ago, I began avoiding pre-packaged, processed foods and started shopping mainly in the fresh produce section of the grocery store. I spent roughly the same amount on food each week and enjoyed the fresh, vibrantly colored, flavor-filled, nutrient-packed meals. When certified organic foods began entering the market they were expensive, so I dug and planted a small organic garden in my backyard. Finding myself perpetually short of time later in my career, I gave up gardening and patronized farmers' markets, health food stores, and any organic farmer who had a food stand. Buying direct made the prices for organic comparable to regular grocery produce. The real bonus was, my family and I were rarely sick.

Today, I spend very little money on doctor visits thanks to two decades of making healthy living a priority. Instead of shying away from paying more for organic produce, I focus on how much "getting the best food sources" *saves me* by reducing health-care costs, lost sick-day wages, and down-time while ill.

What constitutes a healthy diet? Not the Standard American Diet, dubbed "SAD" for a reason. High in simple carbohydrates and sugary foods which spike blood sugar, it is also low in vegetables and healthy fats. The South Beach Diet and Mediterranean Diet are two popular, healthier options. For people suffering from arthritis or other forms of inflammation, however, the anti-inflammatory diet in Appendix B (that follows) outlines the plan I have followed to keep inflammation levels in check.

Why is this important? In my 40s, severe pain in both shoulders kept me from sleeping on either side at night for three years. Because my dad had similar shoulder pains mid-life, I thought it was genetic and thus incurable. But after two months of adhering to this anti-inflammatory diet, all shoulder pain disappeared and has not returned. I still follow it today.

Eat Three Times a Day!

To utilize nutrients effectively, the body needs a wide variety of foods available at the same time. This is why it is important to eat breakfast, lunch and dinner. Kids, people recovering from illness or surgery, and the elderly may also need two small snacks between meals. Each meal and snack should include three different types of food:

- **A variety of healthy carbohydrates,** derived from whole grain cereals (gluten free if needed), breads, beans or other legumes, vegetables, and whole fruits.
- **A variety of proteins,** comprising roughly one-quarter to one-third of a child's meal, from vegetables, soy, nuts, fish, poultry, meats, and dairy (if they digest it properly).
- **Essential omega 3 fats** found in cold water fish, walnuts, flax and chia seed, spinach and dark leafy greens, marine vegetables, and purslane (the 9th most common weed in the world and highest leafy source of omega-3 fats). Omega 6 oils are also essential to health but need not be supplemented, since the Western diet delivers an overload of omega 6s in meats, poultry, dairy products, eggs, and the safflower, sunflower, and soybean oils used for fried or processed foods.

Complex Carbohydrates

Food carbohydrates consist of long chain simple carbs (three or more) linked together, called "complex." Complex carbs also contain vitamins, minerals, and antioxidants. Their fiber slows breakdown and use of foods by the body, thus providing terrific, long-term energy to keep you going. Good examples are green vegetables, potatoes, squash, beans, peas, lentils, and whole grains like oatmeal, brown rice, quinoa,

"Simple" carbs are comprised of one or two sugars. Most breads and baked goods are simple carbs made from processed grains that have been stripped of their natural bran, germ, or endosperm. Softer in texture, they are digested faster, and deliver less healthy nutrients. Sweeteners like table sugar, honey, candy, and sodas are also simple carbs. Easily digested and quickly absorbed, they spike blood sugar and rapidly boost energy. But this energy is short-lived, and unless accompanied by complex carbs may cause blood sugar levels to drop sharply in an hour or two. Although fruits, vegetables, and dairy products are technically simple carbohydrates, because they contain fiber, protein, and other nutrients they act more like complex carbs and should be included in a child's daily diet.

Carbohydrates are great "comfort food." They satisfy by making us feel full. They add pounds, however, if carb intake exceeds what the body uses each day, since excess carbs get stored as fat. Children's needs and metabolism vary widely. As they become more involved in sedentary screen entertainments, it is important to keep carbs intake in balance with protein levels, essential fats, and daily physical exercise.

A child should eat five to nine vegetables *daily*, for their fiber content as well as essential vitamins, minerals, and natural enzymes. Encourage kids to chew their food to avoid choking, and because saliva secreted while they chew contains enzymes that begin breakdown of complex carbs, fats, and starches. All types of carbohydrates are broken down into glucose (blood sugar). Complex carbs take longer and contain important, indigestible fibers that aid gut health as well as regular stool elimination.

Raw fruits and vegetables have an abundance of enzymes that aid digestion, but these enzymes are destroyed if heated above 115 degrees Fahrenheit. This is why serving a small, fresh salad or partially cooked vegetables with meals is customary in many cultures. Lightly sautéed mixed vegetables, accompanied by pieces of chicken, seafood, or meat, and cooked whole grains is an easy-to-prepare, enzyme rich, balanced meal.

A Variety of Proteins

All proteins are made up of amino acid chains. Most people know protein is required by the body to build strong bones, but it is also necessary for making cellular repairs. That scratch on your arm, the muscle you tore - all physical damage is repaired by proteins. Of the 20 amino acids in body protein, nine must come from foods we eat since the body cannot produce them: histidine, isoleucine, leucine, lysine, methionine, phenylalanine, threonine, tryptophan and valine. Arginine is also needed by children.

Some vegetable proteins do not contain all nine essential amino acids and must be paired with other foods to form a "complete" protein the body can utilize. If children are vegetarian or vegan, offering meals and snacks containing complete proteins is especially important. Healthy food combinations that have all the essential amino acids are easily made from beans, lentils, and peanuts paired with whole grains like wheat, rice or corn. A classic example is simple Mexican fare that pairs rice and beans.

Vegans and vegetarians should consider taking sublingual (under the tongue) vitamin B12 tablets daily. Vitamin B12 is crucial for maintaining a healthy brain and nervous system. Yet the highest sources come primarily from animal derived protein: red meat, salmon, mackerel, sardines, milk, Swiss cheese, yogurt, and the "soft" yolk of a 5-minute boiled egg. Vegan sources of B12 are supplements and a few fortified foods: some plant-derived milks, soy products, and breakfast cereals. Mental health is dependent on adequate B12!

Dairy products are an easy protein source, yet they are the second most common allergy among people with mental disorders. (Gluten, the protein in wheat, is the number one allergen.) The least expensive way to determine if food allergies or sensitivities are contributing to mental symptoms is to do an elimination diet.

Remove any food from the diet that results in children or adults becoming tired, cranky, spaced out, or that they consistently crave. After these foods have been eliminated for one month (two months for gluten/wheat testing), serve the food you are testing to the child/adult three times in one day. Over the next 48 hours, write down how their mood and behavior changes. As problem-causing foods are slowly identified, eliminate them from the diet. If you want quick results, order lab testing for food allergies through a holistic medical practitioner or direct from https://www.greatplainslaboratory.com/organic-acids-test-igg-food-allergy-test-candida.

Essential Fatty Acids

Omega 3s, 6s, and 9s are all "essential fatty acids" that the body must have to function but cannot make. Omega 9s are obtained by eating sunflower seeds, hazelnuts, almond butter, macadamia nuts, and foods cooked with saf-flower, soy bean, olive, or canola oils. Americans regularly consume large amounts of omega-6s in meats, chicken, cheese, eggs, nuts, and vegetable oils. We eat far fewer omega-3s because they are primarily found in cold-water seafood, flaxseed, marine vegetation, green leafy land vegetables, and beans, most of which are not the average child's favorite foods. A healthy ratio of omega-6s to omega-3s is believed to be between 6:1 and 1:1. According to some estimates, Americans consume a 20:1 ratio. This imbalance is causing an inflammatory "cascade" inside the body that contributes to the increase in arthritis, heart disease, cancer, and brain disorders.

The brain is 60 percent fat by weight and it is especially dependent on supplies of essential fatty acids to function. Fats are the raw materials used to make cell membranes. Cells communicate with each other through these membranes. The type of fat eaten determines whether the membranes are quick to communicate or slow.

Trans-fats, hydrogenated, and partially hydrogenated oils, such as mar-garine and shortening, are solid fats that can sit on store shelves for months without going rancid. Research by Harvard professor Perry Renshaw, using magnetic resonance imaging of the brains of depressed people, showed con-sumption of solid fats made brain cell communications slower, less responsive. The essential oils, however, are liquid at room temperature and float freely, enhancing cellular communications and brain processing speed.

I experienced the dramatic difference a healthy "oil change" can make. After the causes of my manic highs were identified and halted, 15 months of uninterrupted depression followed, and nobody could figure out its cause. Finally, I heard about Dr. Andrew Stoll's clinical trials, where bipolar patients were taking 10,000 mg of Omega-3 fish oils daily. There was such a marked reduction in their symptoms, the trials were halted half-way through and all patients were put on the fish oils. In Stoll's book, *The Omega-3 Connection*, he recommended adults with mental disorder take 3,000 to 5,000 mg of fish oil daily. I began taking 3,000 mg, 1,000 mg with each meal. To my astonishment, my deep depression lifted just 48 hours after adding these essential fats into my diet in 2002. I no longer experience depression, even during dark, New England winters. (However, I was on an anti-inflammatory diet and taking 1,000 mg of Omega 3s for two years, so improvement time will depend on your diet, toxic load, and how Omega 3 deficient you are.) I now consume fish and seafood three times a week *or* I take 1,000 mg twice daily of high-quality fish oils.

In summary, begin by eliminating all bad trans-fats and deep-fried foods from the family diet. Even if you fry using healthy fats, the high heat of frying damages the fat molecules and converts them into bad fats. Bake, lightly sauté, simmer, or grill foods over low heat instead. If you are depressed or have other mental symptoms, begin taking Dr. Stoll's recommended 3,000 to 5,000 mg of fish oils daily – always with meals. Buy high quality fish oil capsules from reliable sources that have rapid sales. Also check the back label to be sure the oil was filtered for metals and other toxins. (To access lists of seafood having the lowest levels of environmental toxins, go to www.ewg.org/seafood.) Once you start taking the capsules, pay attention to how energetic you feel. The final and most important step is to add *"good Omega 3 fat"* *sources* to your shopping list: avocados, whole eggs, fatty fish, nuts, chia seeds, extra virgin olive oil, dark chocolate, coconut and coconut oil.

Essential Water

People can live six weeks without food but only survive two to ten days without water, depending on the surrounding temperatures and their level of activity. Water makes up roughly 60% of one's weight and is required for all body functions. Water helps maintain our constant temperature of about 98.6 degrees Fahrenheit. It transports nutrients and oxygen to all cells and carries waste products away, while helping maintain blood volume and lubricating both joints and body tissues.

Drinking plenty of plain, filtered, fluoride- and chlorine-free water every day is a great habit. No other fluids are good substitutes. Regular consumption of sugar-laden juice drinks or sodas rapidly elevate blood sugar and contribute to age-onset diabetes. Diuretics, like coffee, tea, and lemonade, release fluids from your system and are recommended only in moderation, not as a substitute for drinking water. The goal is to stay well-hydrated from steady intake of fluids throughout the day, ones that do not dramatically increase blood sugar levels.

A child or teen should drink at least six to eight cups of water a day and eat five to nine servings of fruits and vegetables daily for the vitamins and fluids the contain. Before, during, and after any physical activity, kids need more water, especially in hot weather. Truly the best liquid for maintaining health, water is sugar-free, caffeine-free, and calorie-free.

Exercise and Deep Breathing

Another essential for health is daily exercise. It increases circulation, clears a foggy brain, and helps oxygen flow to the heart and extremities. Daily exercise keeps muscles, bones, and body structure strong. Another reason for exercising regularly is to boost immune function.

The lymphatic system is part of our immune system. It includes tissues and organs that produce and store cells to fight infection and disease. Lymph is a clear fluid carried toward the heart through a network of lymphatic tubes. However, unlike the heart, the lymph system has no pump. Exercise is what keeps lymph moving, carrying debris out of the body during internal housekeeping to maintain a strong immune response.

Research shows group exercise, whether team sports like soccer or backyard games of tag, also fosters neuron development and stimulates hippocampus growth, enhancing both learning and memory. Exercising outdoors, away from traffic and pollution, is shown to rapidly lower stress levels. Even looking at photographs of outdoor scenes reduces stress. To get kids involved, let them choose a favorite sport or exercise. If exercising daily is new to them and they are less than excited after trying their first choice, allow them to choose something else. The objective is to help them discover physical exercise can be "fun" and how great it makes them feel.

APPENDIX B

ANTI-INFLAMMATORY DIET

Eating too much red meat, eggs, dairy, and other foods listed below may cause the body to produce excessive arachidonic acid (AA), a polyunsaturated omega-6 fatty acid found in most animal fats. If excessive intake of AA continues, overproduction of prostaglandin twos will begin as the body attempts to reduce inflammation levels. Unless dietary changes are also made, this "inflammatory cascade" will continue, triggering arthritis and contributing to mental illness, cancer, heart disease, and other degenerative conditions. Often given to patients by Naturopathic Doctors, this diet works to lower the *causes* of inflammation instead of taking pain medications for temporary symptom relief.

Avoid
Red meat
Fried foods, saturated fats, hydrogenated oils
Sugar, artificial sweeteners
Refined foods, flours, and white rice
Dairy products
Wheat products, such as pasta, breads, cereals
Peanuts or peanut oil
Soft drinks, sweetened juices
Coffee, black tea, colas, chocolate
Alcohol
Pharmaceutical hormones
Exposure to herbicides/pesticides and other chemicals

<u>Do Eat, Organic When Possible</u>
Chicken, turkey (free range, antibiotic & hormone free)
Fish (only 2-3 times a week due to mercury and pollutants); limit shellfish
Legumes such as peas, beans, lentils
Whole grains, except wheat
Soy products, such as tofu, tempeh, soy cheese
Eggs, organic and hormone free only
4-9 Vegetables a day, half raw
2 Fruits a day of differing colors
Omega 3 and 9 essential fats and "good" oils from olives, tree nuts, and seeds
Organic dairy products (if not allergic)
Filtered water, herbal teas, green tea, vegetable juices, unsweetened fruit juice
    diluted 50:50 with water

Additional Tips

Eat 4-8 ounces of protein each day (not per meal), depending on your size and level of physical activity. Protein is the primary fuel used for cellular replacement and repair. Animal flesh has a higher percentage of protein than plant sources, so eat a variety of the protein types recommended in Appendix A. Dairy products are a good protein source if testing shows you are not allergic/sensitive to it. But wheat and dairy are the two most common undiagnosed food allergies among people with mental disorders. Food allergies also increase inflammation levels.

Do two "**elimination diets** if you cannot afford allergy testing. Cut out use of dairy products for one month and, in a separate test, eliminating any foods containing wheat/gluten for two months. Keep notes on changes in health or energy during the elimination period. Then eat that food three times in one day, writing down any mental or physical symptoms that appear within 48 hours. If symptoms are obvious, avoid these foods and consider getting the allergies and sensitivities turned off by a holistic practitioner utilizing a Bioset system.

Grain carbohydrates give sustained energy, yet people's needs vary. By eliminating wheat and gluten-containing grains you'll reduce carbohydrate intake and probably lose weight. But do eat gluten-free whole grains, beans and legumes, or you'll be hungry and run out of energy more quickly between meals without sufficient complex carbohydrates.

Eat three meals a day plus two snacks, waiting at least 2-3 hours in between. Each time you put food in your mouth, the body releases insulin, the "hunger hormone." Thus, constant snacking will increase hunger. Only eat nutritious snack foods (vegetables dipped in hummus, bean dips, or guacamole; low-fat cheese; fresh fruits; tree nuts, etc.), avoiding junk and fast foods. Eating small portions of healthy foods five times a day provides cells the fuel required to keep blood sugar, mood, brain power, and energy levels stable.

GRACELYN GUYOL

RECOVERED BIPOLAR PATIENT, AUTHOR,
AND HOLISTIC MENTAL HEALTH ADVOCATE

In 1991, Gracelyn sold her seven-person California public relations agency and retired mid-life to coastal Connecticut with her husband, intending to travel, garden, and play tennis. However, occasional bouts of depression were re-diagnosed as bipolar disorder in1993, changing the course of her life.

An antidepressant was prescribed and life seemed less chaotic, but a year later, the rapid growth of breast cysts and tumors resulted in her having surgery twice in 12 months. Gracelyn consulted a Naturopathic Doctor to help identify and eliminate potential causes of these growths. Cyst development stopped, yet one new tumor appeared. Finally suspecting the drug, she tapered off, and within two months her latest tumor disappeared and new growths ceased. Refusing all psychiatric medications, Gracelyn found drug-free solutions that halted her bipolar symptoms in 2002.

First she celebrated. Then she began writing and speaking to raise consumer awareness of all-natural solutions to mental illnesses. In 2006, Gracelyn authored *Healing Depression & Bipolar Disorder Without Drugs*. She delivered day long accredited seminars to medical practitioners in eight cities in 2007. Her second book, *Who's Crazy Here? With Drug-Free Steps to Recovery* for nine mental disorders, came out in 2010. Between 2012 and 2016, she produced over 40 cable TV shows in an on-going educational series, "Restoring Health Holistically."

Following the 2013 Newtown School shootings, Gracelyn was asked to serve on the new Connecticut Children's Mental Health Task Force, its only member with broad knowledge of complementary and alternative mental health treatments. In 2014, she submitted a recommendation of ten holistic treatments for children's mental problems to the Task Force, which are covered in this book.

In 2017 Gracelyn founded a 501(C)(3) non-profit, Mind Energy Innovations, Inc. Its mission is to: 1) promote holistic, drug-free treatments for mental disorders by educating the public about these options; and 2) sponsor accredited, educational seminars about holistic treatments for medical practitioners to help improve patients access to treatment.

For more information, go to www.mindenergyinnovations.org; www.gracelynguyol.com; and "Holistic Healing with Gracelyn" on Facebook.

Made in the USA
Columbia, SC
18 April 2018